The 2 Week Diet and Detox Plan

The Ultimate Guide to Optimum Weight Loss, Increased Metabolism, and Reaching Your Overall Health Goals

Melinda Rolf

All Rights Reserved. No part of this publication may be reproduced in any form or by any means, including scanning, photocopying, or otherwise without prior written permission of the copyright holder. Copyright © 2015 eQuivia Books™

Introduction

Weight loss and health are not achieved by following a single diet or detox method. What it requires is a thorough understanding of what happens in the body. For instance, weight loss is not just about eating the right foods, detoxification, and exercise. There are many more factors that can influence fat-storage and fat-burning. Many people would agree that even after following strict dietary guidelines and sweating for hours in the gym, they still can't achieve or maintain their weight goals. What could be the problem? They did 200 crunches per day but their muffin tops and love handles still remain. What could they be doing wrong? Should they try a different diet? Do more crunches? What?

The answer is inflammation, metabolism, fat genes, digestion, exercise, supplements and disease-prevention. What do these things have to do with weight loss and health? Read on to find out.

Disclaimer

This book provides general information and discussion about medicine, health and related subjects. The words and other content provided in this book, and in any linked materials, are not intended and should not be construed as medical advice. If the reader or any other person has a medical concern, he or she should consult with an appropriately-licensed physician or other health care worker.

Contents

Chapter 1

A two Week Guide to Health and Weight Loss

Health isn't just about taking good care of a single system. It's not just about the digestive system only or the metabolism alone in order to lose weight, detoxify the body, and achieve optimum health. It's all about balancing everything because every tissue in the body functions only as well as the other tissues.

So, to start your journey to achieving all your health goals, consider going on this 2-week diet and detox process.

Step One: Take measurements

The most important step before starting any health regimen is taking baseline data. Assess the body to see what condition it is currently in. Take body measurements right before starting the diet and detox. This will serve as a point of comparison if the process worked or not and to what extent. Also, depending on current health, a person may need to get some laboratory tests done such as lipid profile, blood sugar levels, urine profile and, in some people, liver function tests. Other important health parameters to take before going on a diet and detox include blood pressure readings, respiratory rate and heart rates.

Step Two: Remove everything bad

Any diet or detox will never work if a person continues to eat the same unhealthy food and live the same unhealthy lifestyle. Before diving into a diet and detox regimen, take stock of what's in the refrigerator, in the pantry, and in the desk drawer at the workplace. Most likely, all the culprits that contribute to all sorts of health issues can be found in these places. Sugary snacks, processed foods, and all other junk foods should be thrown out. Clean these areas first before attempting to clean the body. Otherwise, these will be hard-to-resist temptations that will bring failure to any diet and detox regimen.

Start by throwing out anything that comes in a box, can, or plastic wrapper and was manufactured in a factory. Canned foods are high in fructose and salt, along with a cocktail of other harmful compounds. The same goes with anything in a box or plastic that does not look like real food. However, what may remain in the pantry are canned whole foods such as artichokes and sardines as long as they contain small amounts of artificial ingredients.

Check labels of all drinks. Throw away anything that has added sugar in it. This includes all drinks with artificial sweeteners, cane juice, molasses, maple syrup, honey, and agave. All fruit juices and other beverages sweetened with sugar should also be removed. All sugar-based and flour-based foods should also be removed, especially when they are packaged (candies, cookies, bread, cupcakes, crackers, etc. in boxes or plastic packaging).

All foods that contain additives, preservatives, or artificial colorings should also be avoided. All these can potentially promote health problems. Avoid all foods made with hydrogenated oils, trans fat and refined vegetable oils such as soybean or corn oil.

Step 3: Include the good

Eat only foods that are good for the body. The following chapters will teach what foods are good for specific concerns such as metabolism and digestion.

Step 4: Change your lifestyle

Health is not just about food. It is also about living healthy and taking care of the body. A few simple things that can have a huge impact on health include:

- Getting enough restful sleep – about 7 to 8 hours each night

- Deep breathing exercises for about 5 minutes each day

- Hydration – about 8 glasses of water each day

- Exercise

Chapter 2

Detoxing the Right Way

Detoxification is a natural process in the body, and the primary organ that first comes to mind when talking about detoxification is the liver. But it's not just the liver's job; other organs help too. There are several pathways that the body uses to remove toxins, such as the colon, kidneys and skin. The skin is the largest organ that helps in detoxification. It offers a larger surface area for excretion compared to others, where waste products are removed via the sweat. The kidneys remove wastes from the blood and excrete them through the urine. The colon collects toxins and wastes produced through metabolic processes, packages them with fibers, and then brings them out through the feces.

If any of these exit points is blocked, toxins go back to the cells and accumulate there. For example, if a person is constipated, toxins have nowhere else to go but back inside the body. These can be reabsorbed through the intestinal walls and be circulated by the blood to other organs. This is also why taking adequate water and fiber is crucial to detoxification so that any toxins collected from the body are excreted properly. Water helps promote better movement in the colon. It is also a crucial part of urine and sweat.

Detoxification is a process that heavily relies on nutrients. If done right, the body immensely benefits. If done incorrectly, the body might suffer from more problems that are serious. Most people think that detoxifying means starvation and following a liquid-only diet. It's more than just that. In fact, some of the more popular juice cleanses and starvation-detoxes do not provide the body with the adequate nutrients it needs. So, instead of a real cleanup, the body is placed at higher risk for problems, which can affect hormones and fat control.

Phases of detoxification

A proper detox process has 3 main phases. Phase I involves helping and giving the liver an opportunity to perform its blood-screening function. The liver is the main organ responsible for screening every molecule in the blood. It activates proteins and molecules before the body can use them. It also inactivates those chemicals and proteins that are no longer needed by the body, turning off processes that need to stop. Any toxins and foreign molecules are inactivated, repackaged and tagged for excretion. Some of these go straight to Phase III of detox. Some require further breakdown in Phase II.

Molecules that need further processing before getting eliminated are often bound to molecules such as glycine, sulfate, and glutathione. The resulting compound is now inactive, non-toxic and ready to be eliminated. But, this process produces free radicals as by-products. Free radicals can cause oxidative stress in the body and cause problems. This is where adequate nutrition during the detox period becomes crucial. Certain nutrients are needed to deal with these byproducts and protect the body from any damage.

Nutrient requirement for effective detox

The required molecules to inactivate and bring toxins to the different excretory organs can be obtained from food. These required molecules include enzymes needed for breaking down compounds and antioxidants to protect cells from free radicals and molecules (e.g. sulfate, glycine, and glutathione) that bind toxins. Eat specific foods during detox in order to get these nutrients for detox to be effective. This is contrary to the prevailing misconception that starving one's self is part of detoxification.

There are specific foods to take to fuel each phase of the detox process. It is equally important to eat these foods in the right amounts and at the right time. For instance, eating a lot of foods that promote Phase I but too little of the foods that support Phase II will put the body in trouble. Just like a production line, fast packaging of toxins in Phase I with slow Phase II inactivation and binding will surely back up the toxins and return them to the body.

Phase I key nutrients are calcium, folate, B vitamins (B3, B6, and B12), vitamins A, vitamin C and vitamin E. Great food sources for these nutrients are brightly colored fruits and vegetables, and dark, leafy greens. Soaked whole grains like quinoa are also good sources. Another interesting source is organ meats. On an ounce-per-ounce basis, organ meats bring the highest amounts of some of the needed nutrients for Phase I. such as vitamins A and E, as well B vitamins like B3, B6 and B12. Organ meats are also high in folate.

In Phase II of detox, amino acids are crucial. These include glycine and glutamine, as well as cysteine and taurine. These amino acids are important because they bind with toxins and inactivate them. So, aside from eating fruits and vegetables, you should also consume proteins during the detox process. Without proteins, there will be none of these important amino acids for Phase II of detox. If there are no amino acids/proteins from food, the body will turn to the proteins in the muscles and convert them into the required amino acids for binding to toxins and wastes. This explains why starvation-detox processes produce rapid weight loss. But it isn't fat that is lost. Instead, it's mainly water and proteins. This can be dangerous as losing lots of water (without proper replenishment) can lead to dehydration. Losing proteins from muscles can lead to muscle weakness and atrophy.

Aside from these, effective detox also needs selenium and sulfur. Eggs are a wonderful rich source of sulfur, which is also high in proteins. Other great sources of sulfur are raw garlic and onions. Cruciferous vegetables like cauliflower, cabbage, broccoli and Brussels sprouts also contain sulfur. Fish is a great source of selenium. Brazil nuts are also high in selenium, but should be eaten in moderate amounts.

What detox does

Detoxifying the body has 3 major benefits. It has been scientifically proven that this process help in achieving better control over carbohydrate intake and curbing unhealthy craving for high sugar, high carb foods. Detoxifying revs up the metabolism, too. And, when coupled with the right type of supplement, it can help lose weight.

Controlling Carb and Curbing Cravings

Going cold turkey on bad habits won't work. It can give immediate results but will be difficult to sustain. Experts advise that gradual entry into the process of detox will help in feeling more comfortable and in control. It also helps make the entire process easier and more enjoyable.

During the entry period, the most important step is to avoid foods with negative effects on the body. This includes cutting back on sugar, alcohol, meats, and fructose. Caffeine, dairy and gluten are known to trigger negative reactions such as bloating. It is advisable to cut back on these, too.

Cutting back is done over a few days, typically about 2-3 days. Give the body time to gradually ease off of these things. Otherwise, going cold turkey will cause intense cravings that can lead to greater feelings of deprivation and depression. These feelings are brought about by having to give up on all those comfort foods. Gradually cutting back also helps in minimizing any withdrawal symptoms. This is especially helpful when a person has been consuming these things in large amounts and/or for a long time.

Daily meals consisting of foods with low glycemic index are best for keeping carbohydrate intake under control. This also helps in reducing the sugar cravings. Low glycemic index foods are those that do not cause rapid spikes in the sugar levels in the blood. When blood sugar levels are stable, there won't be any crash (rapid drop in sugar) that usually lead to cravings, low energy, poor focus, sluggishness, etc. The brain signals that create those insistent cravings for sugary foods also stop. Cravings are a huge hindrance to eating healthy and achieving optimum weight. By losing these, making the right food choices will be much easier. And, on the plus side, it will be easier to stick to a healthy lifestyle.

Following a purified, science-based detox involves removing potentially harmful or irritating foods from meals. Examples are gluten and lactose. These food components tend to produce negative reactions in the gut and in the immune system. A significant number of the population is believed to be underdiagnosed, misdiagnosed or underdiagnosed for problems related to these compounds, such as IBD and lactose intolerance. The symptoms are generally brushed aside and inadequately managed, creating more serious problems like bloating and poor weight control. By removing these, most people start to feel better. The removal of the added stress from irritating foods will clear the body and promote better metabolism.

Revving up metabolism

Proper detox is an effective, scientifically-based, and proven method to rev up anyone's metabolism. However, not all types of detox can do this. Some detox methods only remove potentially irritating foods and cause you to lose a little weight. But a few more changes will help in balancing the hormones and promote better health and weight.

Hormonal imbalance is among the top reasons that cause weight gain. This is also among the main reasons why a lot of people who try to lose weight find it difficult to achieve their weight goals. This is especially common among women.

One of the hormones that play a crucial role in weight gain is cortisol. High cortisol levels can put other hormones out of balance. It can block the normal production of thyroid hormones (main hormones driving metabolism) and slow down metabolic rates. Among the main reasons for high cortisol levels include stress, alcohol and too much intake of caffeine.

Estrogen and progesterone levels also affect weight and metabolism. Low levels of progesterone and high estrogen levels increase appetite that can lead to weight gain. Bringing back the levels to normal ranges regulates hunger cues.

An average diet may not provide all the necessary nutrients in the right amounts. Nutrient deficiency makes it harder for the body to make the right amounts of progesterone, thyroid hormones and insulin.

Detox promotes eating more vegetables and fruits. This can help in filling the system with the required minerals and nutrients. However, it may still be not enough. Supplementing can help in giving the body a good boost in revving up metabolism and encourage the body to fat-burning mode. Supplements can help ensure that the body is receiving the needed minerals, vitamins and a few other helpful compounds like antioxidants to swing the body over to a fat-burning machine.

Weight loss

A proper detox may be enough to help you achieve your weight loss goals. Revved up metabolism and eating certain foods can stimulate the body to activate its fat-burning mode. When the body is filled with toxins, the fat storage process accelerates. Fats serve to cover the tissues and protect them from the damaging effects of toxins. Remove the toxins and the tissues will star to shed their fat layers because the threat is no longer there. This will translate to weight loss.

Chapter 3

Understanding the Process of Inflammation

The body is subjected to various stresses and exposed to a myriad of potentially harmful microorganisms and substances. In response to these threats and presence of damage, the immune system responds with an inflammatory response. Inflammation is part of the body's defensive mechanisms. It is a natural response to the presence of threats. However, it is a protective process that, if unchecked, can also cause damage.

How does inflammation happen?

Inflammation is one of the body's intrinsic and immediate responses to any damage or injury sustained by the tissues. The inflammatory response produces the classic set of symptoms: redness, pain, swelling, and heat. The injured or damaged area swells from accumulation of water and other inflammatory chemicals, as well as the increased blood flow. It becomes painful because of the pressure of the swollen tissues on nerve endings. Heat and redness mainly come from the increased blood flow and dilation of the blood vessels supplying the involved area.

The main goal of the inflammatory response is to localize whatever is causing the damage or injury, preventing spread of damage. Also, the effects of inflammation aim to dilute the irritating substance as an attempt to reduce its damaging effects. Then, a chemical process happens in order to inactivate the noxious substance, binding it, taking it away from the damaged area and then eventually excreting it out of the body. After the noxious stimuli are removed, repair and healing can start.

Inflammation is necessary for survival. It isn't a bad process per se, as most people think. Without this, damage, trauma and injuries can easily spread to the rest of the body, wreaking more serious damage.

Stages of inflammation

There are 3 major stages of the inflammatory process. These stages proceed in a sequential manner. If something interferes with the intrinsic regulatory mechanism, problems associated with inflammation happen.

Inflammatory response starts with dilation of the capillaries supplying the site of injury to increase blood flow. The increased blood flow is necessary because immune cells, chemicals, oxygen and nutrients. These are all important in localizing the damage and providing immediate aid to the affected tissues.

The second stage is structural changes on a microvascular scale, along with the proteins in the blood escaping and flowing into the damaged tissues. These proteins play 4 very important roles:

1. These proteins serve as carrier proteins that allow more of the essential elements to enter the damaged tissues for repair and healing.

2. These proteins can help the immune cells to enter the cells of the invading pathogens (if inflammation is caused by microbes).

3. These proteins can provide the necessary building blocks needed for cellular and tissue repair.

4. Some of these proteins can be used as part of the signaling system that regulates the inflammatory process. This stage is also responsible for the swelling that inflammation is also known for. Swelling in the first stage is generally not so obvious, but once plasma proteins start to leak into the area of injury, swelling increases and will become more noticeable. This is because plasma proteins have a strong affinity for water.

The third and final stage is the transmigration of immune cells leukocytes. In this stage, the immune cells pass through the endothelium and accumulate at the site of the injured tissues. Another chemical process is activated once the leukocytes arrive at the injury site.

Basically, inflammation is the first step in a multi-stage immune response to injury and infection. It contains the damage while waiting for the other immune system components to come into play. Also, part of the inflammatory response is informing and activating the other cells and chemicals of the immune system to help out with fighting the trigger and healing the damage.

What does the inflammatory response do to the body?

The main effect on the body after the initiation of the inflammatory response is increasing the blood flow to the affected area. Blood vessels supplying the injury site dilate to allow more blood to flow into the area. Also, the cell walls of the affected tissues open up. Gaps appear in the cell walls, where larger cells like the immune cells can easily and quickly enter. Also, the increase in blood flow to the injured area strengthens the immune action.

Once the immune response is triggered and the inflammatory response is activated, all the other immune cells are summoned and congregate at the site of injury. All these would cause the area to swell, from the increased blood flow, accumulation of immune cells, and the entry of plasma proteins along with the water they attract, into the affected area.

Increase in body heat, particularly at the affected area, is an indication of the intensified immune process that happens. The various chemical processes happening within the affected area generally give off heat as a by-product. More blood rushing to the area also contributes to the generation heat. In itself, heat also contributes to the immune response. Higher temperatures can kill most bacteria. So, in effect, heat functions as anti-biotic effect. Also, heat works in favor of the chemical reactions that the body initiates to protect the tissues from further damage and in fighting off the noxious substance.

As heat increases, the area also turns red. It also comes from the increased amount of blood flowing into the affected area.

Pain happens as the swelling expands. The expansion places pressure on adjacent nerve endings. Another source for the pain is the release of pain chemicals from the damaged tissues. Pain mediators are also commonly activated by the different signaling chemicals that are part of the immune response.

The inflammatory cascade continues until the noxious stimuli or infection has been resolved. In case of infection, phagocytes (cell-eating immune cells) seek the invading pathogen and engulf it. Pus is produced from this pathogen-eating event. This is the leftover debris from the destruction of the pathogen.

How does inflammatory response end?

Inflammatory cascade lasts as long as the invading pathogen or the noxious stimuli is present. Once eradicated, the immune response should end as well. The chemical signals trickle down and eventually stops. The immune cells start to retreat. The blood vessels return to normal diameters and blood flow returns to normal. Plasma proteins return to the blood and the gaps in the cell walls disappear. The cells return to their normal size and the swelling is reduced.

Apoptosis is the main element that ends the inflammatory cascade. This is a unique event where in the involved cell "commits suicide". The involved cell shuts down and stops functioning. Apoptosis in immunity happens when the immune cells no longer receives a signal to remain alive and functioning. The helper T cells are responsible for sending this signal to other immune cells, telling them to continue their immune functions. If the signal stops, these other immune cells "kill" themselves. The helper T cells continue giving the "stay alive" signal to other immune cells as long as they themselves continue to receive signals or detect the presence of antigens (pathogenic microorganisms or noxious stimuli). When infection or trigger is no longer present, helper T cells receive the signal. In turn, they also stop sending the "stay alive" signals to the other immune cells. When this happens, apoptosis occurs in these other immune cells. Thus, this event effectively ends the inflammatory cascade. The body returns to its normal functioning.

What prolongs inflammation?

There are instances when the inflammatory cascade does not effectively end. Three main possible circumstances are widely considered. One possibility is that the infection or noxious stimuli is not yet effectively removed. Either some proteins or leftover segments of the pathogen/antigen/noxious stimuli are still present in the body but the body has no other effective way to deal with it. Sort of like some lint or dirt remains and the body has nothing to clean it up with. Hence, the helper T cells continue to detect its presence and keep signaling the other immune cells to continue functioning. The other possibility is that even when the trigger is no longer present, the helper T cells fail to recognize their absence. A third possibility is that something else is giving the signal to the helper T cell, which prompts it to continue signaling to the other immune cells. This third scenario is often the reason why chronic inflammation develops.

How does inflammation become bad for health?

When the intrinsic control of immune function is disrupted, the originally protective immune mechanism becomes the source of several problems. As a result, the immune system goes out of control.

The body is not designed for prolonged immune function. First off, immune function is meant to be destructive- to destroy the trigger. But, if the immune system remains to function even when the trigger is no longer present, then, problems surface. Either the body's own cells become targets or the effects of the immune process damage the cells. The damaged cells will then provide the trigger that tells the immune system to still continue its processes.

For example, once infective microorganisms are eliminated and the immune process still continues, the body's cells suffer. In inflammation, the continued swelling, pain, redness and heat will cause damage to the cells. Swelling will expand the cells and interfere with tissue functioning. Redness from continued large blood flow will expose the cells to unwanted substances. Remember that the cells form gaps to receive the immune cells. The longer these gaps are present, the more chances that other substances can come in, too. The gaps are like unguarded gates and there is high probability that undesirable substances can enter and cause problems.

What is chronic inflammation?

Inflammation that starts and ends as it should, over a limited period, is called acute inflammation. The process happens when needed and promptly ends when the threat or infection has passed. Inflammation should cease after a few days. But, in some instances, the "off" switch does not work or fail to be triggered. Inflammation and the rest of the immune response associated with it continue to proceed. Chronic inflammation develops.

What started as protective and supportive mechanisms becomes a source of tissue damage. Continued swelling damages the tissues. Large volumes of blood can bombard the cells with too much nutrients and oxygen, as well as other unneeded substances. The events involved in the immune process hinder the normal homeostatic activities. This can lead to all sorts of problems.

A few of the common problems that can arise is problems with cholesterol levels, cardiovascular problems, and problems with metabolism. Triglyceride levels skyrocket. Cholesterol levels become elevated. Fatigue, difficulty in sleeping, low energy, increased susceptibility to infections, depression, and anxiety occur. Overall physical conditions deteriorate and the person manifests dry skin and other signs of premature aging. Chronic inflammation can also cause excessive weight gain and obesity.

How is inflammation detected?

Local signs of inflammation include the 4 classic signs of redness, heat, pain and swelling. But, chronic inflammation can occur without any of these outward signs. A significant percentage of the population is unknowingly suffering from inflammation. Fatigue, decreasing physical health and some other health problems like high lipid profile are often attributed to some other problem. Most people do not consider that these symptoms and health concerns have roots with an immune system that has failed to regulate itself properly.

So, is there any way to check if there is, indeed, hidden inflammation? Despite modern advances in medicine and technology, there isn't yet any definitive test. What remains to be considered as a good indicator for the presence of inflammation is the presence of markers. The highest indicators are the C-reactive protein test and the test for the interleukin 6.

What causes the bad kind of inflammation?

The causes vary. It depends on individual physical constitution and overall health conditions. Some of the known and more common links to the development of chronic (or bad kind of) inflammation includes diet, lifestyle, and presence of certain illnesses.

Lifestyle

Unhealthy lifestyle practices expose the body to harmful chemicals and toxins. For example, sedentary lifestyle can set the body up for poor health leading to inflammation. Lack of exercise hinders the body from effectively metabolizing food and using available energy. Because the body is not using up energy, it is converted into fats and stored. Digestion slows down, causing fewer nutrients to be absorbed. Other chemical processes in the body slow down, too. Poor blood circulation deprives cells of required oxygen and nutrients. Toxins from the various cellular processes build up within the cells. This translates as a threat, triggering immune responses, including inflammation.

Exposure to pollution is also one cause. Pollution can come from the air and/or from water. Toxic emissions from car exhaust and from second-hand smoke are common sources. These enter the respiratory tract and cause respiratory distress. The immune system responds by sending inflammatory cells and chemicals to the lungs, causing greater breathing difficulties. Pollutants in the air and in water can also interfere with the normal chemical signaling pathways in the body, including that of the immune system.

Inadequate amounts of sleep places the entire body out of balance. Hormones are unable to regulate themselves effectively. Immune responses and control become ineffective, too.

Stress is also another cause. It can cause the levels of cortisol to rise and displace all other hormones and chemicals out of control, too.

Diet

Not all foods are good for the body. Some provide good nutrition while some provide empty, unusable calories. Some help improve health while some promote negative reactions. The same can be said when it comes to inflammation. There are foods that contain compounds that worsen or promote the continuation of inflammatory responses that can spell trouble for health.

Trans fat is never good for anybody's health. This a heavily altered type of fat that, when eaten, will trigger inflammatory responses. The structure is something that confuses the body. It contains elements similar to the fats that the body knows to be safe and of use, but there are also some elements that are foreign. So, the body does not know how to treat trans fats. Some are stored as fats (which adds to weight gain and obesity) while some are transported to the tissues in the hope that the cells can find a way to use them. Once in the blood, trans fat can damage the lining of the blood vessels. This triggers an inflammatory reaction. But because of its altered state, the immune system does not know how to properly process the trans fat. Macrophages cannot decide if they should destroy it because of the confusing signals they receive from it. And because trans fat remains in the system, inflammatory cascade continues to occur, leading to problems associated with chronic, systemic inflammation.

The trouble with trans fat is that it is present in a lot of food. It is most commonly found in processed foods. Trans fat is commonly used to prolong the shelf life of foods because the altered fat does not go rancid as quickly as normal, regular, unaltered fats do.

Sugar, specifically refined sugar, is another common food ingredient that is also a common cause of inflammation. First, problem starts with too much consumption of sugar. The body is not designed to be digesting and metabolizing such large amounts. On the average, a person consumes about 22 teaspoons of sugar, about 90 grams per day. But, according to WHO (World Health Organization), less than 5% of the total daily calories should come from sugar. So, for an average 1,200-calorie intake per day, less than 60 calories should come from sugar. A general guideline currently given is 50 g sugar for women and 70g sugar for men. This also depends on the activity per day. People with more sedentary lifestyle should consume less.

The second biggest issue about sugar is the type. There are several forms of sugar available. There are the natural sugars found in whole, natural food. There are also refined sugars. Natural sugars are easily digested and absorbed. The body also effectively uses this sugar type. Refined sugars, on the other hand, are processed. The structure is different from what the body is designed to metabolize. It can't be effectively used. So, the body tends to store refined sugars as fat. In effect, eating more refined sugars translates to more fat storage leading to a bunch of problems like obesity and diabetes. Excess fat can also trigger inflammatory reactions. Fat storage and inflammation spell trouble for the body because one triggers the continuation of the other. As more fat accumulates, inflammation continues, which completes the vicious cycle by stimulating more fat accumulation.

Studies have found that excess sugar in the body has the ability to trigger immune responses, particularly inflammation. Cytokines are activated, which are chemical messengers necessary in initiating the inflammatory cascade.

White bread is another commonly eaten food that is also one of the major causes of inflammation. The effect is the same with sugars. White bread, white pasta and white rice all contain simple carbohydrates that are quickly broken down into simple sugars. These sugars are quickly absorbed by the blood, raising blood sugar levels quickly. In response, the hormone insulin is activated. Large amounts of sugar in the blood would signal large amounts of insulin to be released. The effect is a quick reduction of the blood sugar levels. This would be just fine, a part of the homeostatic process in the body. But, if this happens frequently, like any other thing in life that's too much, problems can develop. The body is not designed to take kindly to constant bombardment of high levels of any hormone, or be exposed to any for a prolonged period. Cells will tune out from the signals they receive from insulin, resulting in insulin resistance.

Rapid rise and fall of blood sugar levels promote the development of unhealthy eating habits. Rapid drop would instantly make a person crave for something high in sugar. This can happen a few moments after eating a full meal. The body recognizes the sudden drop as a threat because the cells need glucose (sugar) for energy. So, even if a person just ate a lot of food, soon, hunger cues are felt.

White bread is rich in refined ingredients. It contains refined grains. Studies have found that refined grains raise the levels of inflammation markers in the blood. Refined grains have been processed and altered too much that it no longer resembles the original structure the body is designed to work with. Hence, like the previous inflammation-inducing foods, refined grains are recognized as foreign substance in the body.

Animal fats have been found to be closely linked to inflammation, based on numerous studies done over the years. These are mostly saturated fats, which can have a huge impact on gut bacteria. Saturated fats can change the delicate balance of the microorganisms that naturally reside in the gut. This change has a significant effect on how the immune system functions. The gut microflora is closely linked to immunity. About 80% of the cells of the immune system are made with the help of the activity of the gut microflora. So, changes in the gut can have a huge impact on immune function. This imbalance has been found to trigger an inflammatory response.

Also, saturated fats contain an inflammation-triggering compound called arachidonic acid. This compound has been found to set off an inflammatory cascade that can go on for a prolonged period.

How the meats are cooked is also a possible cause of inflammation. Cooking with high heat can produce carcinogens. When eaten, these carcinogens can set off an inflammatory response. Using sugary marinades on meats are also possible causes. When the sugar component gets burnt, the resulting compound can trigger inflammation.

The body has use for saturated fats. It isn't some useless, harmful substance in food. The problem only surfaces if saturated fats are taken in large amounts and when cooked improperly. Add this type of fat moderately in the diet to keep the negative effects in check.

Alcohol irritates the gastrointestinal tract. It makes the lining of the intestines more permeable, allowing bacteria from the gut to pass through the bloodstream. Bacteria may be harmless and even beneficial in the gut, but once in the bloodstream, it's a whole different story. It is recognized as a pathogen and will definitely trigger an immune response, starting with the inflammatory cascade.

Another reason why alcohol can induce chronic inflammation is that it is quickly metabolized by the body. Alcohol turns into simple sugars after digestion. This will follow the same pathway as sugars and refined grains go through in the previous discussions.

Alcohol has some positive benefits. It is known to provide some protection against cardiovascular diseases and Alzheimer's. However, if the amount of consumption goes beyond the threshold, any positive effects are forfeited and negative effects become more prominent.

Omega-6 fatty acid is an essential fatty acid. However, the consumption should be at a certain ratio against its relative, omega-3 fatty acid. Omega-6 fatty acid should be eaten in fewer amounts compared to omega-3, but the average meal has the reverse i.e. more omega-6 than omega-3. This imbalance can trigger inflammation.

In simplest terms, omega-6 triggers inflammation while omega-3 lowers it. However, the process is more complex than that. The body has use for both essential fatty acids. They're "essential" after all. But in order for omega-6 to be of benefit, it should be balanced by omega-3. If not, trouble happens. Omega-6 is mostly obtained from some seeds and in vegetable oils.

Milk is a common food either drank on its own or used as a recipe ingredient. It is present in most baked products, as well as in a lot of sauces, dips, gravies, and other dishes.

Milk can be an anti-inflammatory food, but not all forms of milk are good. Low-fat milk can be effective in reducing inflammation. However, whole milk, 2% milk and other milk varieties that contain large amounts of saturated fats that can trigger inflammation. Also, some people are unable to digest the proteins in milk. These people would surely experience an inflammatory reaction to milk.

MSG is monosodium glutamate. This is common in Asian cuisine as a preservative and added flavoring. However, animal studies found suggestive findings that MSG can trigger an inflammatory response. There is little data on how MSG exactly functions in the body, but to be on the safe side, experts caution against MSG use until more definitive research results are available. What is sure is that MSG is not a natural compound. Hence, the body has no natural means of effectively using it.

Gluten is a natural protein common in some grains such as wheat and barley. Some people are sensitive to this. Their digestive tract has difficulties in digesting and effectively metabolizing gluten. This can trigger inflammation in the gut.

Chapter 4

Diet to Reduce Inflammation in the Body

Foods can help in reducing the inflammation anywhere in the body. These foods contain compounds that work in various ways. Some of these compounds inhibit the release of inflammatory signals. Some function by promoting soothing reactions. Some reduce the symptoms of inflammation such as swelling and pain. Some interfere with the chemical signaling that trigger the inflammation. A few others promote healing of tissues that provoke the inflammatory response, while some help in removing toxins and noxious chemicals that trigger the inflammation.

Brightly colored, deeply pigmented

The best foods are vegetables and fruits. The ones that carry a lot of the health-promoting substances are those that have deep colors or the brightly colored ones. Generally, the beneficial compounds are found on the skin, which are also responsible for the bright colors of the vegetable and fruit.

Herbs and spices

A number of herbs and spices are used in traditional healing practices, including the management of inflammation and in the management of symptoms. Examples of herbs and spices with anti-inflammatory effects include turmeric, ginger, garlic, green tea, and oregano. These contain a healthy amount of polyphenols and bioflavonoids that act as powerful antioxidants in the body. These compounds bind with harmful toxins and render them inactive. These bring the toxins into the bloodstream, already harmless, and then to the excretory organs to be excreted out of the body.

Polyphenols and bioflavonoids also limit the production of free radicals in the body. Free radicals may result from some cellular processes, as well as a byproduct of digestion of certain compounds.

Bioflavonoids are also known as flavonoids or flavones. More than 5000 plant chemicals belong to this class of chemical. The body can metabolize flavonoids, which releases active molecules. These molecules serve several functions such as antioxidant, anti-allergenic, anti-cancer, and anti-inflammatory. Some of the popularly known bioflavonoids include OPC's (oligomeric proanthocyanidins), epicatechin and quercetin. OPCs found in grapeseed extract and pine bark extract (pycnogenol) are among the most effective against inflammation. Rutin and quercetin have powerful soothing effects on the inflammatory cascade. Other good sources of bioflavonoids include wine, cocoa, some vegetables, citrus fruits and tea.

Boswellia (Boswellia serrata)

This herb is known also as Indian frankincense. It is part of traditional Indian healing practice, specifically as an anti-inflammatory agent. Scientific studies were performed on this traditional healing herb and found a few interesting things. Boswellia extracts had the ability to turn off the key cell signalers and chemical mediators (cytokines) that support inflammation.

Ginger (Zingiber officinalis)

For centuries, various cultures used ginger as part of their traditional healing practice for several purposes. Modern medicine has started to recognize the health benefits and healing properties of ginger. Pharmacologists and biochemists are now becoming more interested in the various effects of ginger in the body. Some of these include anti-nausea, analgesic, GI-calming, sugar-moderating and anti-inflammatory. Years of research found that ginger effectively works in the same way as NSAIDs (non-steroidal anti-inflammatory drugs). Ginger suppresses the body's synthesis of prostaglandins, one of the molecules that play a part in the inflammatory cascade. This molecule is associated with the pain symptoms of inflammation. A recent study found a promising discovery. Ginger extract shows a strong possibility of deactivating or inhibiting the expression of genes linked to chronic inflammation.

Turmeric (Circuma longa)

This is an ancient herb used for both cooking and healing in South East Asia. In Ayurvedic traditional medicine, turmeric serves as an anti-inflammatory agent. Studies found that the active compound cucurmin has mild inhibitory effects on COX2, a type of pain receptor in the body. It is similar to prescription drugs of a similar nature but does not cause side effects (e.g., increased risk for stroke and heart attacks) that these drugs commonly give. Turmeric also shows indications of effective reduction in joint inflammation. This effect is elicited by initiating cell signaling systems that inhibit prostaglandin synthesis and activate the genes responsible for regulating the inflammatory cascade.

Essential fatty acids

The best essential fatty acid for reducing inflammation is omega-3 fatty acid. The best sources of it are cold-water fishes like salmon, tuna, mackerel, sardines, and anchovies. Shellfish, oysters, and clams are also good sources. However, the health benefits may be negligible compared to the possibility of pollutants in these sources. Waters where these fishes are normally found are also known for high levels of toxins like PCBs and mercury. Experts recommend staying away from fishes caught in Atlantic waters, especially salmon. On the other hand, Alaskan salmon and those caught in the wild Pacific waters are considered safe.

Aside from seafood, other good sources of omega-3 fatty acid are seeds and nuts. Good examples are ground flaxseeds and walnuts. Limit nuts and seeds to only a handful per day because these also contain omega-6 and some other compounds that, in large amounts, can cause a few problems.

Other good essential oils include the omega-6 supplement called GLA or gamma linolenic acid. This is especially helpful in reducing inflammation associated with rheumatoid arthritis. This condition involves an autoimmune disorder that attacks several joints in the body. GLA has been found to effectively reduce inflammation in the joints, suppress the immune system and relieve some of the symptoms.

Omega-9 fatty acid called oleic acid is also effective in reducing inflammation in the body. The most popular item that contains a good amount of oleic acid is olive oil. This can be used for salad dressings or for general cooking. Olive oil is a much healthier alternative to cooking with animal fat or some unhealthy vegetable oils. Grapeseed oil is also a good source. This oil can be used as a healthy oil for cooking. Both these oils are also high in polyphenols that can reduce inflammation.

Strengthening the body's own anti-inflammatory capabilities

The body has its own ability to reduce inflammation. It just takes a few changes in one's lifestyle and activities.

First in the list is to start moving. Exercise is very helpful in improving blood circulation. This can help better substance exchange between the cells and the blood. The waste products of cellular processes enter the blood stream and go to the excretory organs for removal from the body. This prevents the buildup of waste that can trigger inflammation. In addition, good blood flow brings more oxygen and nutrients, as well as antioxidants to the different tissues, strengthening them against any threats. Better blood flow also promotes on-time arrival of chemical messengers that turn the immune process on and off. Another great benefit from regular exercise is for stress reduction.

Lower stress levels in the body improve balance. Hormones are better regulated, as well as the immune response. More benefits are obtained if exercise is coupled with deep breathing exercises. Stress reduction will also help in lowering the chemical and cellular processes that produce free radicals as by-products.

Rest is also very important. A good night's sleep promotes healing, recharging and rejuvenating. Hormones can go back to their normal levels and some of the cellular processes slow down. The body can concentrate more on healing and repairing. Also, adequate, restful sleep can undo the inflammatory effects on the body. During sleep, there is a reduced demand on most of the body's systems, which is taking a huge load off on hormones and immune cells.

Healthier lifestyle also means staying away from harmful activities. This includes staying away from cigarettes or stopping smoking altogether. Recreational drugs like marijuana should also be avoided. If possible, reduce the intake of synthetic medications (work with a doctor on this one). Avoid popping pills like NSAIDs and other over-the-counter medications for everyday aches and pains. Also, reduce alcohol consumption. While studies have shown that alcohol, particularly wine, can have positive health benefits, people who are not drinker should not start. People already drinking should stay below limits on alcohol consumption. Moderate intake can provide positive effects but taking too much will offset these and promote negative effects.

Detox

Detox or detoxification programs help get rid of accumulated toxins in the body. Toxins are like grime that slow down and interfere with normal regulatory processes in the body. By getting rid of it, cells are able to "breathe" and function better.

In truth, no matter how much a person is determined to live a toxin-free and healthy lifestyle, toxins are everywhere. There are toxins in the air we breathe. A few can still find their way in the foods we eat and in the water we drink. No matter how organic whole foods are, it can still pick up a few toxins—whether during transport, handling, or while being displayed in supermarkets. Toxins are everywhere. No matter how much homes are "green" (toxin-free), there will still be pollutants. Green homes reduce pollution but harmful chemicals can still be present—just in much smaller amounts than in "non-green" homes. In offices and in public places, toxins and pollutants are still present. It isn't possible to isolate one's self and live in a toxin-free bubble. People need to socialize and be outside. And in doing so, the body gets exposed.

Toxins are also produced by the body. No matter how healthy the foods are, certain cellular processes will produce waste. And, these wastes can be harmful for health. For example, when the body burns its fat stores, free radicals may be produced. When the body digests proteins and carbohydrates, waste products are formed. All these can be potential toxin sources. These are normal. It is a natural process because not every part of any molecule is usable at all times. The body will just get what it needs at a particular time.

While we can't be totally toxin-free, we can help the body in cleaning itself. Experts recommend undergoing detox about once or twice a year. Give the body an opportunity to rid itself of all the toxins. Detoxifying the body is also a very important step in reducing and eventually treating chronic inflammation. Remember that accumulated toxins can be perceived as threats that can initiate the inflammatory reaction. The immune system will attempt to contain the accumulated toxins within an area and prevent it from spreading and damaging more tissues. This is where inflammatory cascade comes in. As long as toxins are present, the inflammation stays. Remove the toxins through detox and inflammation will surely ease up.

Chapter 5

Understanding Metabolism

Metabolism is a natural body process that refers to all chemical processes within the cells designed to keep the body alive. This is a critical process that keeps the body functioning. Anabolism and catabolism are 2 main metabolic processes in the body. Anabolism refers to "build up" or synthesis of molecules. Examples include when the cells produce hormones, enzymes, proteins, etc. Catabolism refers to "break down" of compounds. The resulting smaller molecules are then used for anabolic processes. Both of these processes require energy in order to proceed.

Factors regulating the metabolic rate

The biggest factor that affects a person's metabolism is the BMR or basal metabolic rate. This is the energy being used just to maintain the various tissues while the body is at rest. About 50% to 80% of daily energy requirement is used for BMR. The energy is used for various activities like digestion and absorption of nutrients (these processes proceed better when the body is at rest), blood circulation, pumping of the heart, peristalsis of the muscles of the gastrointestinal system, hormone production, growth and repair of tissues and so much more.

The top factors that affect the metabolic rate and BMR are age, muscle mass, body size, genetics, gender, physical activity, diet, drugs, environmental factors, and hormonal conditions.

Age can work for or against an individual. Younger people tend to burn energy faster, especially during the growth years. Metabolism starts to slow down after puberty. Generally, people who reach their 30s have slower metabolic rates compared to when they were in their teens and 20s. One of the main reasons is the loss of muscle tissue associated with the aging process. Also part of the slowdown is the natural changes in the neurological and hormonal processes as a person ages.

Muscle mass refers to how much muscle tissue is present in the body. Energy is needed in order to maintain these muscles. Even at rest, the body has to burn energy in order to keep the muscle in a state of slight tension to prevent them from getting flaccid. If there are more muscles, more energy is burned, metabolic rate increases.

Body size affects how fast or how slow metabolism proceeds. People with larger bodies generally have higher BMRs because their bodies have larger internal organs, larger muscle mass, and greater fluid volumes. All these require energy for maintenance. Taller people have wider skin surface areas. That means more surface area for evaporation and cooling. This will require the body to burn more energy just to maintain normal body temperatures.

Genetics also play a significant role. Some people are naturally born with faster metabolic rates compared to others. The presence of certain genetic disorders may also speed up or slow down metabolic rates.

Gender also plays a factor in BMR. Men generally have higher BMR compared to women.

Physical activity can help speed up metabolism. Exercise can help in building more muscle mass and in promoting faster energy consumption. Among the most effective exercises to boost metabolism (with muscle building results) are resistance and strength training like lunges, squats and pushups. Lifting weights also help boost metabolic activities.

Hormonal factors like imbalances can affect metabolic rates. For example, hyperthyroidism can speed up metabolic rates to unhealthy levels. On the other hand, hypothyroidism can slow it down.

Environmental factors like weather can have an effect on metabolism. During winter, the body tends to slow down its metabolic rates to conserve energy, much like hibernating. When the body is exposed to chilly weather, the body burns energy to try to warm itself up. In the summer, the body tends to use a lot of energy in order to keep cool.

Drugs can slow down or speed up metabolism. Nicotine and caffeine are among the most common drug components that can increase the body's metabolism. Use of anabolic steroids and antidepressants tends to promote slower metabolic rates and weight gain regardless of what diet is being followed.

Diet has a profound effect on various organs in the body. It can affect hormonal control, muscle mass, and body size. It can also be a source of speed up or slowdown.

Chapter 6

Diet for Resetting Metabolism

Metabolism can slow down due to aging, the type of diet, lifestyle, illnesses, and exposure to harmful toxins. It also slows down as part of the normal aging process. Regardless of the prevailing conditions, there are a few things that can be done to reset metabolism and bring it back up.

Making changes in the diet

The diet has to change. It has to change into something other than the current one because obviously, it's not working out well. This means removing a lot from the current diet. Dietary changes have to be sustainable, and for a diet to be sustainable, foods have to be healthy but still palatable. Foods should also be easily accessible, easy to prepare, and affordable.

Sticking to a healthy diet that revs up metabolism requires willpower. Nobody has a lot of willpower all the time to stay away from delicious, delectable, tempting food. Keep these 3 things in mind to help strengthen your resolve to change your diet into a healthier one in order to reset your metabolism.

> *Prepare and eat most of your meals at home.* This is critical in order to accomplish 2 main things. First, preparing and eating meals at home allows for greater control on what types of foods and ingredients will make it to one's plate. One particular issue that requires control is intake of salt and sugar. These are 2 of the most common ingredients that can have a huge impact on health and prove to be a challenge to monitor, especially in the case of food prepared by someone else. Second, preparing food at home helps one avoid situations that make it difficult to stick to a healthier lifestyle. For instance, steer clear of certain restaurants since their menus are filled with tempting dishes that aren't always healthy.

> *Prepare foods in the simplest way.* Foods should stay as close as possible to their natural state even after cooking them. This way, the nutrients remain as intact as possible. Examples of proper preparation would be grilling and baking. Stay away from unhealthy cooking methods such as deep-frying. Experts do not recommend cooking with extremely high heat as this can destroy nutrients and possibly produce harmful chemical by-products.

Load up on proteins and fiber. To restore normal metabolic rates, eat more lean proteins and fiber. Half of the meal plate should have lean proteins such as scrambled eggs, chicken breast and sirloin steak. The other half of the plate should contain vegetables rich in fiber. Protein and fiber help to feel full faster and more satisfied with the meal. These nutrients take time before they become fully digested, which helps to stave off hunger longer.

Even with these 3 key elements, there is still a chance of failing. Home cooked foods may still cause a few problems if one lacks knowledge on what to eat and how to prepare healthy foods. For instance, weight gain will continue even if you cook and eat at home if your meals are low in fiber and high in fat and in calories. Examples include pasta, white breads and white potatoes. Processed foods or processed ingredients may cause problems as well. Home cooked foods will require more than just taking the time to prepare everything from scratch. It also requires knowing more about what goes into the plate. It takes dedication, time, patience, and perseverance for this to succeed.

Carbohydrates and metabolism

These nutrients play very important roles in determining health and metabolism. Carbohydrates, in particular, are a huge driving factor when it comes to blood glucose levels and insulin action. The type of carbohydrates in food can be for good or for bad. Bad carbohydrates can contribute to the development of a big belly, and a big belly may be a sign of insulin resistance.

Bad carbohydrates are those that trigger unhealthy spikes in blood sugar and insulin levels. These are easily digested and rapidly absorbed. Rapid rise of sugar levels in the blood trigger the immediate release of a large amount of insulin in order to restore normal levels. The rapid rise and fall of sugar levels may seem good at first. But, the brain interprets this is a threat. Rapid decline may be interpreted as starvation or that the body has increased need for energy. In response, the brain will trigger hunger cues, driving the person to eat to supplement the falsely perceived increased need for energy.

Insulin will keep acting on these sugars in blood, promoting the storage of excess sugar as fat. And, for some reason, these are more often stored as belly fat. Over time, the cells refuse to respond to insulin.

The accumulating abdominal fat contributes to the hormonal problem. These fats secrete small amounts of hormones that promote further fat storage. Abdominal or belly fats are also resistant to burning. Anyone who has ever tried to lose weight and burn fat would realize that one of the hardest to get rid off is belly fat.

When the body has insulin resistance, metabolic inflexibility develops. This problem can be managed by just making better choices when it comes to carbohydrate intake. Reducing carbohydrate intake can help in decreasing and regulating insulin levels in the body. Studies have shown that even a small drop in the amount of insulin in the blood can already initiate a large improvement in metabolic rates. This can also greatly increase the body's rate of fat burning.

Going on a low-carb diet does not simply mean strictly restricting carb intake. In fact, restricting carb intake excessively may do more harm in the long run. Too little intake of carbs may be interpreted by the body as starvation mode and lead to fat storage rather than fat burning. It is important to take just a little below the daily carbohydrate requirement to stimulate fat burning and avoid initiating starvation mode.

When to eat carbohydrates is just as important as what type of carbohydrates to eat. There are 2 best times to enjoy carbohydrates during the day: breakfast and after working out. Starting the day with a good breakfast of healthy carbohydrates will provide easy to use and easily accessible glucose. Carbs will be instantly burned and used throughout the day, leaving little to be stored as fats. Good carbohydrates for breakfast include steel-cut oatmeal and other whole grains. Another best time to get carbohydrates is immediately after a workout. Eating carbohydrates like a baked potato can help in refueling the body after an exercise routine. Carbs are immediately used instead of getting stored as the muscles recover from the strain of the routine.

Intermittent fasting

Intermittent fasting is not eating for at least 8 hours, once or twice a week. The main goal of intermittent or short fasting is to "force" the body to burn fat stores for energy. If the body is well fed round-the-clock, it will develop the tendency to rely on immediate food for energy. Any excess gets stored as fat. When more energy is required, the brain will send a signal to eat in order to fill that energy requirement. Stored fat/energy remains untouched. By going on short fasts, the body is sort of reminded that there is a stash of energy just waiting to be used.

Everyone can benefit from a fast, even those who have stubbornly inflexible metabolisms. The body gets that much-needed push to start using some of the fats stored in various places within the body.

First-time fasters should manage their expectations and start moderately. Some beginners find it easier to extend the natural fast that happens during sleep by skipping breakfast. The body isn't eating during sleep, so the body is naturally going on a fast at night. Take this example:

9pm dinner;

Sleeping for 8 hours (at 10PM);

Wake up at 6AM the next day

This person would have already spent 9 straight hours on a fast. Easy, isn't it? However, during sleep, a person might not be burning enough of the fat stores for BMR activities (e.g. repair, breathing, and digesting). In order to push the body further and ensure that some of the fat stores do get burned, you should skip breakfast to extend the fast. This way, the body will have to burn fat stores to provide energy for the body to use during the entire morning before energy from lunch meal becomes available. However, skipping breakfast on a regular basis is not highly recommended. The body will suffer from not having enough energy in the morning, leading to sluggishness and to an even lower metabolic rate to conserve energy.

Some people prefer to eat early dinner as a means of extending fasting during sleep instead of skipping breakfast. The short fast is broken by a regular breakfast. However, some people find themselves awake in the middle of the night, hungry and unable to go back to sleep. Find a schedule that works for one's lifestyle and unique needs.

Another better option for those who find the fasting periods difficult is to start small. Try to have a 6-hour interval in between main meals. One simple method is to eat breakfast at 6AM, lunch at 12PM, and then dinner at 6PM. Vary the times as long as there is at least 6 hours in between main meals. Then, as the body is able to adjust to this schedule, increase the intervals. If the body can tolerate, try to fast for an entire 24 hours once per week. If not, then follow an easier fasting schedule.

Fasting won't be easy. There will be struggles, such as discomfort, low energy, and intense cravings, but the body will benefit much from fasting. The body will be able to adjust to fasting periods and things will be much easier the longer one devotes to intermittent fasting. Soon, it will be easier to fast for longer periods and reap more benefits.

Intermittent fasting is only successful if the person will still follow a healthy diet. All the pains of going on a fast will be for naught if the fast is broken by eating unhealthy food like fast food and processed snacks.

Chapter 7

Understanding Fat-Controlling Genes

Look around you and notice how people's body shapes are different. There are people who naturally have large bodies that no matter how much they exercise and starve themselves, or how healthy their lifestyle is, they don't seem to lose weight. Some can eat anything, mostly unhealthy food, and have no exercise but have slim bodies. Fat distribution varies, too. Some people are overweight, but their bellies are relatively flat. Most of the fat deposits are on their arms and thighs. These people are often classified as having pear-shaped bodies. Some are slim, but their middles have accumulated fats. This body type is often called an apple-shaped body. The reason is genes.

Fats in the body

Advances in science and research technology paved the way to the discovery of genes that control how much fat is made in the body and where these fats end up. But before delving into these genes, understand the natural state of fats in the body.

Types of fats

There are basically 3 types of fats in the body: white, brown, and brite. White fat cells are created by the body directly from food. Excess nutrients from food, specifically sugar, are converted into fats and stored in different areas of the body. White fat cells are highly resistant to burning. These are difficult to mobilize and to be converted into energy. Studies have observed that white fat cells have a high tendency to get stored over the belly area. Several studies found that people who are overweight tend to have more white fat cells in the body.

Brown fat cells are fats stored in the body that can get easily converted into energy. It is quickly burned to supply the body's needs instead of getting stored. These are often seen close to the different skeletal muscles in the body. For a long time, brown fat has been thought to be present only in babies. These were believed to provide insulation as the baby's own thermoregulatory mechanism is not yet fully established. Brown fat in babies is believed to give them the necessary energy they need in order to survive during the early days after they are born. In 2009, research has found that adults can also have brown fat in the body. The name is a reference to the reddish-brown color of the fat tissues when observed through a microscope. This unique color is due to the abundance of blood vessels surrounding the cells and the large number of mitochondria within the cells.

Brite refers to the intermediate color of this third type of fat cells in the body. It is a condensed form of "brown in white." This is because these act like brown fats as they are quickly burned and converted into energy. This is what piques the interests of the scientific world and gives a glimmer of hope into the issue of obesity. Preliminary studies have shown that burning white types of fat cells turns them into brite fat cells. Once converted, the body burns these instead of storing these.

Fat-controlling genes

Recent studies have found a few genes that influence fats in the body. Most of these genes translate (i.e. carry information that creates) into proteins and hormones that act on different tissues and organs. Once activated, these hormones, organs, and tissues influence fat activity. Studies and breakthroughs in the field of genetic research found at least 3 genes that show a huge promise in accurately predicting where fat will eventually end up.

So far, research has identified genes that produce 3 main hormones in the body, namely, leptin, ghrelin and neuropeptide Y.

Leptin is commonly called the obesity hormone because of its substantial effect on fat storage. This hormone is produced mainly by the fat tissues. Its function is to act as a thermostat in the body, regulating the body's need for energy. The leptin threshold varies among individuals. Some have high leptin threshold while some have lower. When the levels of leptin fall below the body's set threshold, the brain interprets it as starvation. It signals other tissues to conserve their fat stores. The individual feels hungry and prompted to eat. More often, because starvation is considered a threat, the food choices are towards those that contain high levels of readily available energy – high-carbohydrate, high sugar foods. Then, these foods are quickly converted and stored as fats. Generally, leptin should help in protecting the body from shortage of energy.

If the body starves and the need isn't promptly supplied, the body is forced to burn its precious fat stores, even the ones that protect the vital organs. This can expose the sensitive organs to trauma, friction and injury. Fats act as cushion, a protective pad around organs to prevent them from being seriously damaged from mechanical (physical) pressure. It also acts as a gatekeeper that keeps compounds in the blood from easily entering the cells.

If inadequate calorie intake continues, the body will be forced to metabolize the stores within the muscles. It sort of "digests" the muscles in order release the glycogen stores and convert them into glucose for energy. Once the body starts burning energy stores in the muscles, severe problems develop. The body is on a steady decline, leading to muscle wasting and death. Leptin prevents this from happening, ensuring that the body will still have fat stores that can supply energy whenever needed.

When leptin resistance develops, "fat-storing" mode is promoted in the body. The body fails to recognize the proper leptin signals. High leptin levels mean that the body has enough fat stores. Failing to read this signal leads the body to continually seek foods high in quick energy and then rapidly storing them as fats. Fats accumulate and the body remains on fat-storing mode. Hunger cues are felt more frequently than normal, leading to frequent eating and compounding the problems. Also, leptin resistance makes it harder to burn the fats. Even if the person regularly and properly exercises, the fats refuse to be mobilized and burned. All these factors lead to weight gain and obesity.

Ghrelin is another hormone made by certain genes in the body. This is referred to as the appetite hormone. Higher ghrelin levels prompt the body to seek satisfaction or reward by eating. As a person eats, the ghrelin levels gradually decreases leading to satiety.

However, some factors influence ghrelin levels to remain high, prompting the body to seek out food in order to feel better. One factor is sleep. People who are sleep-deprived have higher levels of ghrelin compared to people who had a good night's sleep. The ghrelin levels tend to remain high despite eating. This explains why people who do not get enough sleep are more likely to become overweight.

Neuropeptide Y is among the numerous chemicals that regulate brain functioning. In the brain, this neuropeptide (brain protein) is believed to influence appetite, possibly in relation to changes in stress levels and mood. It is also believed to increase the body's rate of converting food calories into fats and storing them.

Fat control process in the body

The entire fat control process is like a thermostat. There is a set point that keeps the entire mechanism working as it should in order to maintain weight. When calorie intake is low, the fat-regulatory mechanism slows down metabolism and increase appetite. These responses are designed to slow down fat burning and to regain any fat stores that may be lost. On the other hand, when calorie intake is high (as in overeating) the fat regulator raises the metabolic rate to burn the extra calories. Appetite is reduced to discourage adding more calories to the body.

Several factors can disrupt the natural fat control process in the body. These factors cause the body to produce more fat and resist any attempts to burn them. For example, rapid spikes in blood sugar levels and the resulting false perspective of potential sugar/energy shortage override the fat-control mechanism. Appetite suppressant function of the fat-control mechanism fails to work. Efforts to burn the fat stores are perceived as a threat to the body's emergency energy stores. It becomes more difficult to burn fats and the fats accumulate at an accelerated rate.

Sugar and fat-control

Sugar is the single greatest factor that can trigger the body's internal fat control mechanism. For years, fat from foods have been blamed for excess weight. Recent researches found otherwise. It's actually sugar.

Fat does play a role in weight gain, but sugar is the one that determines how fast the body creates ad accumulates fat. Fructose, in particular, can activate the body's fat-accumulation switch. This results in the loss of normal appetite control mechanism and in the reduction of metabolic rates. This type of sugar interferes with the normal signaling systems in the body, overriding the natural control and promoting an insatiable appetite and in increased fat accumulation.

Fructose can be found in large amounts in foods that contain HFCS or high fructose corn syrup. Another major source is table sugar or sucrose (formed by the combination of fructose and glucose). HFCS are commonly added to processed foods in order to enhance their flavors and to serve partly as preservative.

One interesting thing that happens when a person eats sugar is the increase in the production of uric acid. When uric acid increases in the body, the liver and the intestines have better sugar-absorbing abilities. This sets the body up for weight and sugar problems. The intestines become more permeable to sugar, leading to higher blood sugar levels. The liver becomes more accommodating to sugar. It converts sugar into fat and stores it within its tissues. Excess sugar from the increased absorptive capacity also gets deposited as fats to different parts of the body leading to obesity.

It is crucial to stop this process early. Clinical observations showed that when the body has enough time to adjust to the higher capacity to metabolize fructose, a higher set point for fat is produced. When this happens, it becomes a challenge to restore it to its lower levels. High fat set point increases the rate of fat accumulation, insulin resistance, higher levels of triglycerides, and elevated blood pressures. This process also initiates a low-grade inflammatory process. With sugar-induced obesity, more serious chronic diseases may also develop, such as aortic aneurysms, strokes, congestive heart failure, and coronary artery disease.

Chapter 8

Disable Fat-Storing Genes

The fat set point has to be challenged and restored to its lower, normal, and more functional levels. For this to happen, fat-storing genes have to be deactivated. These steps can help in disabling the genes that drive fat-storage.

Increased physical activity. This is a natural and effective method of reducing the fat set point in the body to allow fat burning. The best exercises that help push beyond the body's fat set point and effectively burn more of the fat stores are combination exercises. Routines should combine aerobic low intensity exercises with anaerobic, short-burst, high-intensity activities.

Low-intensity exercises enable more oxygen to enter the cells, improve blood flow, and tone the muscles. These generally do not require too much effort. All it requires a person is to engage in activities that increase breathing rates to a maximum of 10 breaths per minute. That means no real panting and sweating during or after the exercises. This type of physical activity includes easy biking, swimming and walking.

High intensity, anaerobic, short burst exercises help in strengthening the heart muscles, increasing muscle mass, improving lung capacity, and burning fat. Examples are interval sprinting and resistance training. These activities are known to increase the metabolic rates that continue to remain high for as long as 24 hours after the exercise has already ended. Another good example is progressively accelerating cardiopulmonary exertion training routine. It can effectively turn the fat-burning switch with just a daily 10-minute exercise.

Healthier meals. To turn the body on fat-burning mode, stick with whole, simple foods. Avoid anything that has a long ingredients' list. Estrogenic foods should be avoided, too. These foods contain small amounts of estrogen that can disrupt the hormonal balance in the body. These foods include sesame, dark beans, flax seeds and soy, among others. These foods may also produce inflammation that can lead to obesity and other chronic illnesses.

Eating enough good fats and proteins stabilizes blood sugar and insulin. These nutrients are required in the synthesis of important hormones. Eating too little of these can cause hormonal deficiencies because the body has too little to work with.

Supplementation. Proper supplementation can further help the body in burning fat more efficiently. One of the few good supplements is omega-3 fish oil.

Cut back on sugar

Cut out sugar, specifically fructose, in order to switch of the fat genes. The recommended daily sugar intake should not exceed 4-5 teaspoons a day. In fact, the lower the intake, the better. The body can still create glucose (energy) from other nutrients like carbohydrates and, at times, proteins and fats. Added sugars should be limited and should come from natural sources like those found in fruit.

Avoid artificial sweeteners or processed (refined) sugars. The best way to cut out a large percentage of added sugars is to stop drinking fruit punches and soft drinks. The effects of fructose on the body are not only related to the concentrations, but also the frequency and rate. That means that negative effects will still develop even if just drinking small amounts of sweet beverages on a daily basis.

Natural sources of sugars are acceptable. Because they are natural, the body is able to metabolize and use them efficiently. Natural sugar sources are also rich in healthy compounds like vitamins and antioxidants. These can help in blocking the negative effects of added, unhealthy sugars.

Cut back on carbs

The body can convert other food nutrients into sugar. One of the biggest sources is carbohydrates. This is why it is equally important to reduce intake of the bad types of carbohydrates because these can induce the same negative cycle that bad sugars do. Refined or white carbs must be removed from the diet because they are just as bad as fructose.

Controlling carbohydrates requires better understanding of this nutrient. The body uses carbohydrates as a major source of energy. Removing or severely restricting intake can lead to more weight problems because it will induce starvation mode. The requirement is keeping carbohydrate daily intake to 25-30% of total calorie intake.

One key to successfully avoiding carbohydrates from getting converted into fats is to schedule it properly. Restrict carbohydrate intake for 2 of the 3 main meals of the day. That means eating carbs for only 1 meal per day. This way, the body can fully utilize the carbs to provide for the energy requirements. This is also why most experts recommend eating carbs for breakfast and then eat vegetables, fruits, meats and fats for lunch and dinner. Carbohydrates in the morning will be effectively converted into energy to fuel the day's requirements.

Foods that turn off the fat genes

Aside from limiting the 2 most important compounds that influence the fat genes, there are some foods that can also help in regulating these genes for better health and weight goals.

Dark chocolate

Mitochondria are small organelles inside every cell. The number varies depending on the function of the cell. For example, cells that work harder and longer have more mitochondria than cells that perform relatively smaller functions. Cell mitochondria also have crucial roles to play in controlling fat production. If more mitochondria are activated and given the needed fuel to function, the cells themselves can regulate fat production.

Dark chocolate is known to replenish mitochondria in the cells. Eating about a quarter of a chocolate bar containing 70% cocoa each day is believed to be enough to produce desirable effects. The compound flavinol, particularly epicatechin, blocks a lot of the effects of sugar (fructose) in the body, as demonstrated in a study involving mice. In this same study, epicatechin also shows high potential in stimulating the cells' mitochondria. This can be helpful in enhancing cellular function and improving muscle mass.

One study done at the Louisiana State University found that microbes in the gut ferment dark chocolate, releasing compounds that have anti-inflammatory effects. These compounds also exhibit some protective and supportive effects on the heart and blood vessels. These substances also demonstrate capabilities in shutting down the genes that are linked to inflammation and insulin resistance.

Oatmeal

Oatmeal is rich in fiber, which has loads of functions in the body. Fiber acts like a sponge and binds with toxins in the gut. It also attracts fats, making them less absorbable through the intestinal walls. By incorporating oatmeal into daily meals, people can experience about 25% reduction in the total cholesterol levels. Blood glucose levels may also drop by as much as 10%.

Fiber is also needed in creating bulk in the intestines, which helps in regulating peristalsis and promoting regular bowel movement. Toxins should be eliminated from the body on a daily basis because the longer they sit in the intestines, the more chances these have of crossing the intestines and joining blood circulation.

The best time to get oats is in the morning. To amp the benefits, you should add fruits to oatmeal. Fruits are also rich in insoluble fiber, the same fiber type in oatmeal. This type of fiber feeds the healthy bacteria in the intestines. Bacteria in the gut are known to produce a very important compound, a fatty acid called butyrate. This is a potent compound that reduces inflammation in the body that contributes to the activation of fat-accumulating process. One study in Canada also found that eating more insoluble fiber promotes higher levels of ghrelin, which translates to better hunger control.

Red vs. green fruits

To turn off fat genes, the best fruits to eat are red ones. The red color is due to the presence of the bioflavonoid anthocyanin. The redder the color of the fruit, the higher the amount of anthocyanins. This particular bioflavonoid has a calming effect on genes that promote fat storage. Phenolic compounds in red stone fruits (e.g., plum) also have a modulating effect on fat gene expression.

Guacamole

Avocados work wonders on belly fat. This fruit may be difficult to incorporate in the diet but making them into guacamole is a great way to eat more of this wonderful fruit. Avocados are rich in monounsaturated fats. These compounds help to reduce the frequency of hunger cues. Another benefit from avocados is that the unsaturated fats show some preventive effects in the accumulation of fat in the belly area- the most common fat storage and area and very difficult to get rid of.

Plant proteins

Proteins are very important in everything. These are needed in the activation and in the control of various genes, enzymes, hormones and all other cellular processes that occur in the body at any given time. Protein is needed for growth, repair, and maintenance. It is also crucial in regulating the fat genes.

Some people prefer to take protein shakes to provide their daily protein requirements. However, most protein shakes bought in the market are filled with a long list of chemicals. These added chemicals can potentially upset the gut and can cause bloating and inflammation. Another concern is the presence of whey protein in these commercial protein shakes. Whey is added to boost the protein content. In high doses, whey can disrupt gut balance and cause bloating.

Plant proteins can be used instead of whey and commercial protein shake mixes. It provides the same benefits such as fat burning, hunger control, and muscle building, but without bloating and other GI discomforts.

Eggs

Eggs are small, simple and unassuming but pack a mighty powerful mix of nutrients. They are rich in proteins, vitamins and healthy fats. Eggs are also the most versatile and easy-to-use nutrient delivery system.

Eggs are the primary source of an important nutrient called choline. The action of choline in the body is to inhibit the action of the genes that trigger fat storage around the liver. Fat accumulation in the liver can lead to all sorts of problems, such as liver disease and poor detoxification of the body. Choline is also found in collard greens, seafood and lean meats.

Citrus fruits

Aside from high levels of vitamin C, citrus fruits contain a potent antioxidant called delimonene. This antioxidant is present in large amounts in the peel. It stimulates the liver to release more enzymes that will flush out more toxins from the body. These liver enzymes also stimulate the intestines to move in a normal rhythm. To get most of the delimonene in the fruits, prepare "detox water". Wash different citrus fruits like grapefruits, oranges and lemons. Slice them up and soak them in a pitcher of fresh, clean drinking water. Sip this throughout the day for an all-day detox.

Nuts

Different nuts, particularly peanuts, are rich in resveratrol and genistein. These 2 compounds can effectively inhibit the action of genes for fat storage. Genistein is a compound that can directly influence the genes responsible for obesity. It inhibits the expression of these genes and reduces the body's fat-storage capabilities. Lentils and beans also have genistein.

Wild salmon

Cold-water fishes like salmon are rich in lean proteins and beneficial omega-3 fats. The lean proteins fight fat accumulation and boost metabolism. When buying salmon, choose the ones caught in the wild instead of the farm-raised variety. These farm-raised fishes are commonly available at local supermarkets and may have been fed with substances that can cause problems in the body. Wild salmon caught in cold waters (from areas free from mercury pollution) are much healthier and provide more health benefits.

Cold-water fishes pack a lot of omega-3 fatty acids. Approximately 1,253 mg of omega-3 and only about 114 mg of omega-6 are present in wild salmon. Farm-raised salmon have 1,900 mg of omega-6 and only a few milligrams of omega-3. The ratio of omega-3 and omega-6 in wild salmon is beneficial because the body can get the omega-6 benefits without triggering inflammation. But with farmed salmon, the higher concentrations of omega-6 can trigger inflammation and fat storage, with only a meager amount of omega-3 to tame down the inflammation from omega-6.

Leafy greens

Watercress, collard greens, arugula, kale and other leafy green vegetables contain a fat-busting compound called sulforaphane. This compound targets the genes responsible for the differentiation of adipocytes (fat cells). By influencing the genes, sulforaphane can influence stem cells on what type of fat cell they will turn into- more towards the healthier type.

Chapter 9

Improving Digestion

The digestive system is another important system that can affect overall health. Poor nutrition, absorption, and bowel movement all contribute to toxin buildup and illnesses. Poor motility results in constipation. Wastes are not regularly removed from the body, which gives these bad compounds greater chances of crossing the intestinal lining and enter the blood. Other negative effects of poor digestion includes weight gain, difficulty losing weight, poor immune function, low energy, and increased risk for diseases to name a few.

To improve digestion and improve health, lifestyle and diet changes are crucial.

General tips on improving digestive function

Improving the function of the digestive system immensely helps in keeping the body healthy. Simple ways to bring back the natural rhythm include eating fiber, getting hydrated and performing regular exercise.

Fiber

Fiber is a very important food nutrient that directly influences bowel movement. This is mainly obtained from plant food sources. The body cannot digest and use fiber but it has very important actions. It attracts toxins and wastes and binds them for excretion.

There are 2 types of fiber in plants. One is soluble fiber. As the name implies, soluble fibers can be dissolved by water in the gut, forming a gel. This gel has several functions including deactivation of dissolved wastes and toxins, ease of passage of stool and protective coating to the intestinal lining. Soluble fiber can be obtained from beans, oats, apples, peas, barley, carrots and citrus fruits.

The other type is insoluble fiber. This does not dissolve in water and forms a major portion of the bulk of the stool. Adding more of this type promotes regular bowel movement and prevents constipation. Both soluble and insoluble fibers help in reducing levels of cholesterol and bad fats in the body.

Water

Water is vital for health. It helps to flush out toxins, promote hydration and improves absorption of nutrients. In the gut, water combines with fiber to form bulk in the stool.

Water also has an integral role in proper breakdown of nutrients during the entire digestive process.

Drink at least 8 glasses of water each day (approximately 2 liters). In warmer weather, when exercising or ill, you should drink more. People with larger body size also have higher daily water requirements.

Watch out for signs indicating that the body needs more water. Signs include sweating very little even when hot or performing strenuous activities, feeling lightheaded and/or nauseous, and feeling unusually tired in the evening. Also increase daily water intake if the urine looks darker or when urinating less frequently than usual.

Probiotics

Gut health is heavily influenced by bacterial colonies normally residing in the gut. Eating food containing cultured healthy bacterial strains can help to support the healthy population of the beneficial bacteria in the gut. These bacteria help in digesting certain nutrients better, promoting more nutrients to be absorbed by the body. These bacteria also help in defending the gut and the body against pathogenic microbes. The best thing about probiotics is that the benefits are not limited to improving digestion. It also promotes better health conditions of the heart, the immune system and the rest of the body.

Vitamins

Essential vitamins are important for a number of reasons. These are needed by the various cells in the body, including those in the GI tract. The presence of vitamins like vitamin A, D, B and C help in metabolizing nutrients such as fats, carbohydrates and proteins better. These vitamins also help in the absorption of certain minerals. For instance, vitamin C enhances the absorption of iron and vitamin D increases the absorption of calcium in the intestines.

Exercise

Exercise is not just for burning fats and building muscles. It also helps promote better digestion. Physical activity helps in strengthening and improving muscle function, including the function of the muscles that line the entire gastrointestinal tract. It promotes normal contraction of these muscles, promoting better churning and digestion, as well as passage of food and stool.

Timing meals

When to eat is just as important as what to eat. For most people, a daily routine may involve eating 3 large meals—namely, breakfast, lunch, and dinner—but some people may find the need to eat in between the scheduled meals. Some people may also find it hard to digest large amounts of food at one time. These people may do better by eating smaller meals spaced throughout the day compared to eating 3 main large meals. This meal schedule can also be used to control the cravings and the need to eat in between main meals. The smaller amount of food may also lessen the stress on the digestive system.

When eating, eat slowly and chew food well. Bigger chunks of food are much harder to digest than smaller ones. Just think of the difference between how a food processor grinds food when bigger chunks are placed into it and when smaller pieces are put in. Bigger chunks make it harder for the food processor to grind food properly. That's pretty much how digestive system works.

Eating too fast also interferes with proper digestive process. It's like bombarding the food processor with a lot of ingredients all at once. It won't be able to properly grind up all the food, resulting in a mixture of properly ground bits with larger chunks of food instead of a perfectly consistent mixture. Eating fast also does not give enough time for the stomach and the brain to communicate effectively. Stomach stretch receptors are stimulated in the presence of food. A signal is then sent to the brain, which would translate to feeling full. If a person eats too fast, the brain still thinks the body is hungry even when in truth there's already a lot of food in the stomach. This contributes to overeating, as well as poor digestive process.

Follow daily meal schedules. Avoid eating meals at random or at inconsistent hours like eating breakfast at 6 AM one day and then 9 AM the next. Following regular meal times helps to train the body to anticipate food and start preparing for it. For example, if the body is used to eating breakfast at 7 AM, the gastrointestinal tract starts to release digestive enzymes and peristalsis quickens. It's like warming up the machine so that when food comes, digestion can start immediately.

Avoid eating right before going to sleep or late at night. This often results in heartburn or acid reflux. The esophageal sphincter relaxes when it's time for bed. Gastric juices can go up and irritate the esophageal lining. Stimulating the release of the gastric juices late at night tends to produce too much of these digestive juices, which can also contribute to heartburn.

Healthier lifestyle

Lifestyle can negatively affect digestive function. For example, smoking triggers hyperacidity and cause heart burn. The lower valve of the esophageal sphincter may get damaged by the harsh chemicals in cigarettes, worsening heart burn and promoting more serious problems like ulcer and cancer. Even those who are exposed to second-hand smoke may suffer as well. Also, exposure to exhaust and air pollution can set off this same negative effect in the body. Steer clear of smokers (or quit smoking) and avoid any prolonged exposure to areas with heavy air pollutants.

Reduce stress

Stress can interfere with the digestive system in many ways. First, high levels of stress promote increased production and release of digestive juices. This can promote irritation and damage to the lining of the GI tract. It can also cause acid reflux and heartburn. Constipation may also develop with chronic high stress levels, along with diarrhea, weight gain and poor immunity. It also increases the risk for GI ulcers.

Ways to reduce stress include getting a massage, performing yoga, taking relaxing baths, and meditation. Exercising is also a good way of reducing stress. The endorphins (feel good molecules) released during exercise can help in relaxing the body and reducing stress.

Chapter 10

Foods for Digestion

Foods affect how well the digestive system functions. Some may irritate the gut and promote poor digestion. Some help relieve any irritation and promote better motility.

Worst foods for digestion

Fried and fatty foods

Foods with high fat contents and fried foods can irritate the gut. These foods often promote the development of heartburn and acid reflux. The bad kind of fats also promotes poor gastric motility and poor digestion. It can lead to steatorrhea, a condition characterized by poor fat absorption, pale-colored stools with excess fat in them. It can also trigger digestive problems such as IBD (irritable bowel syndrome). Avoid fried foods and those that have high fat contents such as cream and butter.

Processed foods

These are the worst food for the gut and for health in general. Most processed foods are high in calories (which the body cannot efficiently use), high in fat, and have loads of artificial compounds that set off negative reactions in the body. Artificial compounds in processed foods promote slowed digestion and constipation.

Aside from the added artificial substances, processed foods tend to have large amounts of unhealthy types of fats and sugar, along with large quantities of salt. These 3 are a potent mix in promoting poor health and impaired digestion.

Chili peppers

Some people may benefit from chili while some may be too sensitive to the potent compounds in spicy foods. In large amounts, chili can be irritating to the lining of the digestive tract. The compounds in chili and other spicy foods can trigger pain and inflammation, leading to poor digestive function.

Dairy

Milk, cheese, and other dairy products are excellent sources of calcium needed for health, but the lactose content may irritate the lining of the gut. A lot of people are having trouble digesting this molecule, a condition known as lactose intolerance.

Experts believe that a number of the population suffer from lactose intolerance without knowing it. The symptoms of bloating, cramps, diarrhea and gas may have been mistakenly attributed to some other reasons. By continuing to eat dairy, more serious damage may result, like killing off good bacteria in the gut.

Alcohol

Alcohol has a relaxing effect on muscles when taken in moderate amounts. This could also relax the muscles of the digestive system. However, you should exercise caution when consuming alcohol since relaxation of the esophageal sphincter due to alcohol intake can lead to heartburn. Gastric juices can easily go up the esophagus and cause a burning, painful sensation. This can irritate and damage the lining of the esophagus, which is not designed to withstand the highly acidic nature of gastric juices.

In the stomach, alcohol can cause an inflammatory reaction. It can impair the action of certain digestive enzymes. This can also prevent the absorption of vital nutrients because alcohol competes with absorption. The irritating effect of alcohol in the gastrointestinal tract can also cause cramps and diarrhea.

Moderate alcohol intake may give benefits, especially on the cardiovascular system. The general guidelines for moderate alcohol consumption are a maximum of 2 drinks for men in a day and for women, no more than 1 drink. But individual reactions are best gauges. For those who are not used to drinking alcohol, experts advise avoiding alcoholic beverages altogether or else more harm may come than good.

Berries

Berries are packed with antioxidants and are generally good for health. But experts recommend avoiding certain berries. Moderate consumption is highly advised for berries with tiny seeds. The hypothesis is that these tiny seeds may trigger irritation and inflammation. These seeds are believed to potentially obstruct the tiny pockets within the gastrointestinal tract.

Chocolate

It isn't actually the cocoa but the milk in most chocolate bars. People with milk allergies and lactose intolerance may suffer from inflammation due to the presence of milk in chocolate treats. Another potential source of irritation is the caffeine content of cocoa. Caffeine may cause diarrhea, bloating and cramps.

Yogurt

Yogurt is filled with live cultures of healthy bacteria that can improve gut microbial balance. Restoring microbial balance is very important to regulate GI function and improve overall health.

Kimchi

This is a traditional Korean dish made from fermented cabbage and spices. Sometimes it also contains onions and radishes. Cabbage promotes healthy bacterial growth in the gut, which improves digestion. Cabbage is also rich in insoluble fiber that further improves the digestive function. However, kimchi is more commonly available in a very spicy flavor, which can irritate the GI tract in sensitive people. Look for non-spicy varieties instead.

The best foods to improve digestion

Food can be used to improve digestive function. These nutrients have various functions in the gut. These can soothe inflamed, irritated lining of the gut. Some can stimulate normal gastric motility and promote regular bowel movement. Some improve bacterial populations in the gut and improve digestive capabilities.

Lean proteins

Proteins are important in digestion. Instead of eating red meats (which are a lot fattier), choose leaner meats like fish and chicken. Lean proteins are also lined to lower risk for colon cancer compared to red meats.

Fibers

These are crucial in promoting better digestive function. Great sources of fiber include whole wheat bread and foods made with whole grains like brown rice and oats. Daily fiber intake should be around 20-30 grams.

In the gastrointestinal tract, fibers reduce bloating, cramps and gas, but these same symptoms may be experienced if one eats too much fiber too soon. You should instead slowly and gradually include fiber in the diet until you have reached a comfortable level of intake. For those suffering from gluten sensitivity, avoid fibers from wheat grains.

Bananas

These simple fruits can help in restoring normal bowel rhythm. Bananas are especially helpful in people suffering from diarrhea. This fruit can help restore potassium and electrolytes lost through loose, frequent stool. Potassium is also a very important mineral in muscle function. It can help in restoring normal muscular movement of the GI tract. Fiber is also present in bananas, which helps to create bulk and restore the normal quality of stool.

Ginger

For thousands of years, ginger has been used worldwide to promote better GI health. It is a safe and effective method of relieving nausea, loss of appetite, colic, motion sickness, vomiting and morning sickness.

Ginger is very effective but should be taken in moderation. Studies have found that taking around 2 to 4 grams of ginger per day can lead to heartburn.

Bone broth

This homemade, delicious broth can help in improving digestion. It is simple but nutritionally dense. It is packed with minerals that help improve health. It also has gelatin (from collagen in the bones) that has a soothing effect on the gut. It is rich in glycine and proline, which are amino acids that improve the function of the gut.

Chapter 11

Understanding Stress in the Body

Stress isn't always a bad thing. Like inflammation, stress is a normal response designed to help the body survive. The problems only start when stress reaches high levels and continues for a prolonged period.

Causes and sources of stress

The first step to understanding and beating stress is to determine its origin. Basically, everything is a potential source of stress. It can come from the maintenance requirements of the body, from daily activities, exposure to the environment, work, career, studies—in other words, pretty much everything. The most common and constant sources of stress are instances such as death (of a family member, significant other, friends, etc.), crime (being a victim of a crime or social injustice like mugging and burglary, etc.), family issues (divorce, etc.), and all other major life-changing events. Career and work environment are also major triggers of stress.

Body response to stress

When subjected to stress, the brain's hypothalamus sends a signal to the adrenal glands to produce stress hormones designed for fight-or-flight responses. These hormones are cortisol and adrenaline. Both of these hormones are highly effective in supporting the body through the stress period. It increases heart rate and breathing rate, as well as blood pressure to ensure that the tissues get what they need like oxygen and glucose to function well in time of greater need. Once the source of stress is gone, the stress response should stop. Levels of adrenaline and cortisol should also decrease.

The digestive system also experiences changes in response to stress. The body needs more glucose as fuel for the increased body requirements. The liver works more in order to produce more glucose. The digestive tract slows down in times of stress because blood flow is diverted to other tissues. This means that fewer nutrients are obtained from food. More pressure is placed on the liver to produce glucose to supply the increased energy requirements. Muscular action is more on skeletal muscles and not on smooth muscles like the ones found along the gut.

The muscles in the body tense up. It is a natural survival response that aims to protect itself against injury. Tense muscles are also quicker to respond and act accordingly to match the body's needs. These are essential part of stress response for survival.

Symptoms of stress

Stress affects the entire body, but some people are not aware of the damage stress is making in their body. Most people are not aware that stress is a risk factor for serious chronic illnesses like cardiovascular problems, diabetes, stroke and cancer. Common symptoms of stress include emotional issues, physical problems, cognitive difficulties and behavioral changes.

Emotional changes related to chronic high levels of stress include:

- Moodiness

- Easily becoming frustrated and/or agitated

- Feeling overwhelmed

- Feeling no control over what happens in life

- Difficulty in calming, relaxing or quieting the mind (thoughts are racing)

- Feeling bad about oneself, depressed, or lonely

- Feeling of worthlessness

- Avoiding social interaction

Physical symptoms of stress include:

- Low level of energy throughout the day, even right after waking up

- Frequent headaches

- Muscle complaints such as tenseness, pains and aches

- Increased heart rates

- Chest pains

- Sleep problems like insomnia

- Increased susceptibility to infections and colds

- Decreased performance or desire for sex

- Grinding teeth and clenched jaws

- Difficulty swallowing, dry mouth

- Sweaty or cold feet and hands

- Ringing in the ears

- Nervousness and shaking of the hands

Cognitive symptoms of stress include:

- Racing thoughts

- In a constant state of worry

- Poor judgment

- Disorganized and forgetful

- Difficulty to focus on one train of thought or activity

- Pessimistic

Behavioral symptoms include:

- Appetite changes, eating more than usual or eating less

- Avoiding responsibilities and increased procrastination

- Increased intake of alcohol and drugs, increased use of cigarettes

- Exhibits nervous behaviors such as pacing, fidgeting and nail biting

Effects of chronic, high levels of stress

Stress affects the body in various ways. Some people may be surprised by how much damage stress can bring to the mind and body, as well as interfere with normal daily functioning.

Stress and emotions

Stress can make it difficult to keep emotions in check. A person under high levels of stress can easily fly off the handle. They easily lose their cool and snap at people around them. Even the most mild-mannered person can suddenly become snappy and hotheaded when under constant stress.

One recently conducted study was able to determine that even at mild levels, stress can make it more difficult for a person to control their emotions. The study also taught stress-relief techniques to the participants. Then, their hands were dunked in icy water to stimulate mild levels of stress. Pictures of spiders and snakes were then shown to the participants. Observations found that these participants were unable to control their fears and anxieties, despite knowing techniques on how to reduce their stress levels. This shows that people have trouble with using cognitive techniques to cope with stress, even at mild levels, such as stress from normal daily living.

Stress and diseases

It has long been established that stress increases a person's risk to develop certain diseases. In fact, chronic stress is a risk factor in several chronic, serious illnesses such as cancer, liver cirrhosis and fatal accidents.

Stress and your love life

Yes, stress can interfere with love life. Sex is a good stress buster but it can also zap the fun out of it. One study found that stress can interfere with libido by wreaking havoc on hormones (particularly testosterone) and affecting sexual performance. Stress increases anxiety and interferes with thought processes, in turn interfering with enjoyment and performance. It can also cause weight gain that interferes with physical the balance of hormones that regulate sexual drive. Stress is also linked to the development of impotence.

Stress and teeth

Habits related to chronically high levels of stress can lead to poor dental health. Highly stressed people tend to have clenched jaws and grind their teeth, even while sleeping. This can wear out the teeth and the jaws can get out of alignment. These people are also less focused, forgetting to perform personal hygiene well. Saliva of highly stressed people also changes in relation to high levels of stress hormones. Saliva tends to become too acidic, which can lead to accelerated erosion of the teeth enamel.

Stress and the heart

The heart muscles can get damaged due to stress. The stress hormones stimulate the heart muscles to work harder in order to increase the heart rate. Stress hormone also acts on blood vessels, causing extensive constriction. Constricted blood vessels make it harder for blood to flow. In response, the heart is forced to beat harder and faster to push more blood through the narrowed vessels. This is a normal adaptive response in order to ensure that enough blood reaches the different tissues in the body. Like all tissues and machines, the harder the heart works, the quicker it fatigues. The muscle tissues wear down much quicker, too. All these increase a person's risk for heart diseases such as stroke and heart attacks. This phenomenon also causes blood pressure to rise, creating more health problems.

Stress and weight gain

Stress is perceived as a threat to the body, triggering survival mode. Part of the survival mode is to pile up fats in the body. Higher levels of stress hormones trigger fat storage and inhibit fat burning. Also, people who are under stress tend to eat more. It's because the body is sending signals to eat more, especially those that are high in calorie and sugar, in order to provide more energy to sustain stress responses.

Stress and aging

Stress makes a person look older. It is a contributory factor to premature aging. On the molecular level, stress shortens the telomeres (terminal portions of the chromosomes/DNA). Shortened telomeres are molecular signs of aging that will translate into poor protein production. This then results in symptoms of aging such as poor skin elasticity resulting to wrinkles, poor collagen synthesis resulting in weak bones, etc.

Stress and the muscular system

Tense muscles are helpful in survival mode, but muscles are designed to contract only for a short time. They need to relax and recover before they can contract again. The length of recovery depends on the type of muscle, but every muscle needs ample time for relaxation. If not, then injuries can happen.

Pain is most common sign of stress affecting the muscles. The most common painful muscles are those over the shoulders and back. These tight muscles can reduce blood flow to the brain, causing frequent headaches. General body aches are also very common.

Stress and the immune system

Response to stress is part of the survival mechanism that seeks to preserve the body and to protect the organs from potential damage. It is a response to both good and bad experiences. Stress is necessary because it keeps the organs functioning well. What makes it bad, dangerous even, is when it is in moderate to high levels for a prolonged period. Recent studies have also found that even mild levels of stress for a prolonged period can also be bad.

When subjected to stress, the heart rate increases. Breathing rates also increase, to supply more oxygen and to release carbon dioxide (produced as by product from cellular processes). Basically, these changes help the body in times of stress. It's like running an engine a bit faster in order to flush out any accumulated grime and to discourage sludge to form. But, stress response is meant to be for short-term only. Prolonged stress will produce various problems.

The severity of these effects depends on how long the body has been subjected to stress and the levels of stress to which it is exposed. To avoid these health problems, start making changes in your life as early as now. That includes making time for exercise, getting rid of unhealthy habits, and making changes in your diet. It also includes learning how to deal with and reduce stress.

Chapter 12

How to Reduce Stress

Stress has to be dealt with effectively and kept under control in order to harness its good benefits and keep the negative effects under control. Avoiding chronic high stress levels include learning stress-busting techniques, exercising and eating right.

Activities to reduce stress

Living a healthier life and learning how to relax are keys to controlling stress levels. Exercises like walking and strength training can help in getting rid of stress. These can also help in promoting better hormonal balance, oxygenation and blood flow that helps reduce negative effects of stress. Exercising also stimulates the synthesis and release of brain chemicals that promote relaxation and feeling good about one's self.

Other stress-busting techniques are meditation, deep breathing exercises, getting enough sleep, taking time to get away from stressful situations (e.g., taking vacations, time-outs or simply spending a few minutes in a quiet room), and yoga. Spending quality time doing enjoyable activities like hiking, sports and some hobbies can also help bust stress.

Foods that reduce stress

Food influences different bodily functions, including how the body deals with stress. Some foods have powerful compounds that help balance hormones, strengthen the body and reduce the negative effects of stress.

Avocados

This fruit is packed with B vitamins, which are known for supporting nerve cells and brain health. It can help relieve emotional symptoms of stress such as anxiety. Avocados are also rich in potassium and monounsaturated fats, which can help reduce elevated blood pressures in times of stress. Eat avocados whole or make into a delicious, creamy guacamole. Try to include them in fruit smoothies or slice them up and add to fresh salads.

Leafy greens

When stressed, people are more likely to eat unhealthy foods like greasy burgers, French fries and sugary snacks. But, these will just increase stress. Instead, grab something green. Munch on fresh green salad that has a lot of leafy green vegetables like spinach and lettuce. Leafy greens are rich in folate. This compound can be used by the body in producing dopamine, which is one of the body's feel-good brain chemicals. A few studies demonstrated improved mood and energy levels when eating green leafy vegetables, suggesting that this type of food can help improve how the body deals with stress.

Turkey breast

Turkey is rich in tryptophan which is a protein that helps in regulating hunger. It is also used by the body in producing serotonin, a brain chemical associated with feelings of well-being and happiness. One study demonstrated that people who took tryptophan had better emotional control and are more sociable. Aside from turkey breast, other rich sources of tryptophan are eggs, beans, lentils, tofu, oats, seeds, fish and nuts.

Oatmeal

Oatmeal is a good source of healthy carbohydrates which the brain also uses to make serotonin. Eating oatmeal is a better choice when cravings strike during stressful times. The brain tends to look for carbohydrate-rich food in order to have more raw materials to produce serotonin and improve mood. Instead of reaching for unhealthy sugary foods, opt for oatmeal. It contains complex carbohydrates that the body can use in its own stress-reducing process but won't contribute to the stress-induced high blood glucose levels.

Yogurt

Gut bacteria plays important roles in stress response. And taking better care of the gut will help in better stress response. One study found that the probiotics found in yogurt can effectively help in reducing the brain activity in the areas handling emotions and stress. This can help in reducing stress signals from the hypothalamus, reducing the body's stress response.

Salmon

Stress can increase the anxiety hormones like cortisol and adrenaline. Omega-3 fatty acids can help in reducing negative effects of stress such as inflammation. The damages brought about by stress eventually become stressors themselves. In reducing these damages, stressors are also reduced. Studies have shown that people who took omega-3 experienced significant reduction in their anxiety levels. Salmon and other cold-water fishes have high omega-3 fatty acid contents. One serving of salmon, about 3 pounces, contains as much as 2,000 mg of omega-3, enough to reduce anxiety and stress, as well as other health benefits like cardiovascular protective effects.

Blueberries

This fruit is high in phytonutrients and antioxidants which are compounds that help the cells fight free radicals released due to stress. Studies have found that blueberries have a lot of helpful compounds that trigger the release of natural killer cells. These cells are part of the immune response that are vital in fighting off stress.

Pistachios

Phytonutrients in pistachios promote better cardiovascular health, reducing any negative effect due to stress. Also, these nutrients have antioxidant action that promote better stress-busting actions.

Chapter 13

Lose the Belly Fat Naturally

Belly fat is one of the most stubborn fats in the body. A lot people may have already achieved their weight loss goals but their belly fat remains. Some people look fit with beautifully toned arms and legs, and yet their belly fat refuses to go away. The explanation lies in the nature of belly fat.

Understanding belly fat

When the body starts to store fat, the belly is one of the first areas where fat accumulates. This is also the last part to give up its fat stores.

Belly fat has protective functions. The belly area is where vital organs of the digestive system is located. It is not protected by the ribs, which makes these organs vulnerable to traumatic injuries. The organs are only protected by muscles. To reinforce the protective layer of muscles, fats stack up. So, basically, the body views belly fat as a vital protective structure- one that it won't easily give up.

While it has supportive and protective functions, too much belly fat can cause problems. These fats have hormone-producing capabilities that create hormonal imbalance in the body. This imbalance promotes more fat accumulation in the belly area and anywhere else in the body. A larger waist circumference due to belly fat is also linked to serious health problems like cardiovascular diseases and type 2 diabetes.

How to burn belly fat

Burning belly fat is not about doing as many crunches as possible. It takes a more intelligent approach to working out in order to bust those stubborn belly fats.

Stop the crunches

Crunches do target the core muscles and strengthen them. But, it isn't the hard-and-fast rule to follow to burn belly fats. Doing 200 crunches a day will not burn those fats because spot reduction is just a myth. It helps but it isn't the entire solution.

In fact, too many crunches can cause more troubles and do very little to belly fat. It can cause pain in the lower back, and promote a forward head and slouched shoulders posture.

Strength training

Get stronger with strength training as it builds more muscle mass. Remember the discussion about muscle mass and metabolism- more muscle mass, higher metabolic rates to maintain these muscles, more fat burning and less fat storage. Strength training also prevents muscle loss and promotes fat loss instead. One of the best exercises in strength building is doing deadlifts and squats. The natural posture for this routine keeps the back straight, with the lower back in the upright position the entire time. The abs are also stretched, promoting more energy burning from the muscles. Both the muscles in the abs and lower back work during deadlifts and squats, preventing collapse during the entire routine. It also works out all the muscles in the body, from head to toe. Fast muscle building and strengthening occurs. The abs muscles are strengthened and the waist size is reduced.

Start with low intensity

Start fat burning mode with low intensity exercises involving aerobics and weight training. This is very helpful for those who have a lot of excess weight to lose. This reduces the amount of strain and stress that the body is exposed to at an early stage. Then, gradually increase intensity as the body is starting to get used to the idea of exercising and fat burning starts.

Moderate intensity aerobics can burn a significant amount of body fat is done right. It should at least keep the heart rate up at most 70% more than baseline. Also, extend moderate intensity routine to more than 30 minutes per session.

Weight training

For weight training, doing more reps (repetitions) using moderate weights is more ideal for beginners than going for fewer reps with heavy weights. As the body starts to burn the fats, start adding more weights and then reduce the repetitions. High reps with heavy weights can potentially cause injuries. Also, when weight training, focus on routines that target the larger muscle groups. Routines that also exercise various muscle groups at the same time are recommended. Another great thing about weight training is that it revs up the metabolism and keeps it up for as long as 24 hours after a session. That means continued fat burning and muscle building even after the training session has ended.

Walking

Walking is for everyone and for every health goal. This is low impact, low to moderate intensity and highly effective. Spend about 15 minutes to an hour to work out various muscles at the same time.

Healthy eating

Eating right is also part of reducing belly fat. All your hard training will be for naught if your meal plate continues to be filled with junk. Avoid all junk foods as well as processed foods and ingredients. Aim to eat the following proteins, fruits, vegetables and the good type of fats and carbohydrates. Good protein sources are plant proteins, eggs, lean meats, fish, poultry and cottage cheese. Good veggies are the green and leafy ones like kale, spinach and broccoli. Great fruits for better muscles and for burning fat include pineapples, bananas, apples, pears and oranges. The good kind of fats includes olive oil, real butter, fish oils and oils from seeds and nuts. Good carbohydrates are those found in oats, whole grains, brown rice and quinoa.

Alcohol should be limited. Despite all the studies that say alcohol is great for health, take it in moderation. Those who do not regularly consume alcohol should not consider adding it into their daily routine. Avoid drinking sweetened alcoholic drinks and beer too often. Notice that men who drink too much beer have pear-shaped bodies with the so-called "man boobs" and abundant belly fat.

While there are good carbohydrates, it does not mean eating an unlimited amount. Anything in excess gets stored as fat. Lower carb intake so that the body will be forced to burn fats to meet the energy demands. Most fitness experts recommend most of the day's carbohydrate allotment after a workout. This way the body burns the calories as soon as they are released into the blood.

Avoid starving

Starvation will not promote fat burning. Instead, it promotes fat storage, with higher resistance against fat burning. Starving one's self means there's less energy for the body to use. That would mean poor performance in work and daily responsibilities. That also means less energy for exercising. When exercising or performing strenuous activities while starving, the body will burn muscles for instead of fat. What results is a skinny body with fats especially around the middle.

Proteins are very important, especially when trying to lose belly fat. These are tough nutrients, and require more energy in order to be fully digested. This is called thermic effect- the body has to burn more energy in order to properly and efficiently process proteins. Compared to carbohydrates and fats, proteins have a higher thermic effect. So, eating more proteins means burning more calories. On top of that, proteins help to feel full and satisfied with meals early into the meal, and these feelings lasts longer. This means getting hungry less often than when eating carbohydrate-rich meals.

Fats are important to burn fats. If the body has a healthy supply of fats for its various needs, then it won't have to store any. One of the best ones to take on a daily basis is fish oil supplements that contain a good amount of omega-3 fats. Start this daily regimen by taking 6g per day.

Healthy eating at a glance

Here's a set of simplified healthy eating rules to follow to blast those fats:

- Eat breakfast.

- Eat light and nutritionally packed snacks or meals every 3 hours.

- With each meal, incorporate fruits, vegetables and proteins.

- Carbohydrates should be taken after a workout.

- Drink 2 glasses of water at each meal.

- Eat about 90% of whole foods for each meal.

- Add cardio exercises to your daily routine.

- Measure your body fat with a caliper every 2 weeks to check your progress. Measurements do not have to be accurate. This is just a better tool to see progress because merely looking at the belly or at the body in the mirror is not a reliable indicator. Images can be distorted due to light, type of mirror, etc.

- Measure your waist circumference and check how your clothes fit. These are great motivators as you notice your clothes starting to fit you better.

Chapter 14

Meal Plans for Health

A carefully planned meal is a sure way to getting on the road to good health. Whether aiming for weight loss or for improving bodily functions, meals should be well-thought out and carefully planned. A good meal plan keeps one on track and reduces incidences of reaching for unhealthy snacks or buying fast food takeout for lunch or dinner. A meal plan also lessens the need to have to make food choices at each and every meal.

To keep things easy, here's a practical sample menu. For each meal, there are 14 different choices. The menu plan is presented as follows to allow for combination choices instead of a menu plan for one entire day. It's like a menu at a restaurant where the diner gets to choose what to eat for appetizer, main and dessert instead of being presented a set menu for an entire meal.

Breakfast

Breakfast is the main and most important meal of the day. But, it does not have to be very heavy with huge batches of pancakes and large servings of eggs and bacons. It has to be packed with nutrients and energy to last the whole morning. It should be nutritionally dense and not just calorie-rich. Fruits are best to provide the vitamins and antioxidants to jumpstart metabolism for the day. Proteins are often most recommended to be from plants, like seeds and nuts, instead of from animal like the traditional bacon. Eggs are also good sources, along with non-dairy butters.

Sample menu

Choose from any of these examples of power-packed breakfast options:

- Power smoothie: This is very versatile because anything nutritious can be tossed into a blender and whipped up to a smooth consistency. Drink in gulps and the body's is set for the entire day. Toss different kinds of fruits with a few greens. Instead of milk or cream, add nut milks like almond milk. Try using coconut cream, too. Fruits serve as natural sweeteners, but do not overdo it. It's better to add just a few slices of fruits and more of the vegetables. Add some seeds like chia seeds for some crunch.

- Omelets: These are easy to prepare and very versatile. Like with power smoothies, anything can be tossed in an omelet to make a nutritionally-packed breakfast. Sauté some starchy root crops like diced carrots and sweet potatoes, along with colorful vegetables like bell peppers. Top with cheese before eating. Meats can also be sautéed and then added to omelet to increase proteins.

- Quinoa: This is a versatile whole grain that's perfect for breakfast. This can be eaten much like oatmeal.

- Oatmeal: One of the healthier breakfast staples is oatmeal. Top with berries or fruit slices for a more complete breakfast meal.

Do not forget to start the day with a few glasses of water. Fitness experts recommend drinking a glass of water to start the day. This helps to wake the different organs in the body and jumpstart metabolism and keeps it up throughout the entire day.

Lunch

Lunch should be filling but not "coma-inducing". Some people load up on carbohydrates for lunch and then spend the rest of the afternoon in a sleepy state. To avoid this, choose to have fibers and complex carbohydrates that keeps metabolism up but will also keep energy up for the rest of the afternoon. For this, vegetables are best.

Sample menu

To get more vegetables and complex carbohydrates for lunch, try these lunch options:

- Salads: The perfect way to get a variety of vegetables in one meal is to make salads. Get a warm salad of boiled root crops, blanched vegetables like asparagus and broccoli, and wilted leafy greens. Or you can have some fresh salads made with crunchy greens like lettuce, tomatoes, cucumbers, carrots, and celery. There are so many options when making salads. Blanch fresh vegetables, pickle them, grill, steam, sauté in nut butters, or bake. Drizzle with a tablespoon or two of olive oil or make some dressings. Instead of using cream for dressings, use coconut or almond milk. Or, use Greek yogurt. Make some vinaigrette with red wine vinegar and olive oil. The options are endless.

- Proteins: Lunch proteins are essential to ensuring a steady supply of energy throughout the afternoon and to reducing the mid-afternoon sugary snack cravings. Grilled chicken, slices of pork tenderloin, turkey breast, and some beef are good choices of protein. Some may prefer to get plant proteins at this time of the day because there is an entire afternoon to digest the tough proteins. Try beans in burritos or with fresh salad. Tofu is also a great plant protein source.

- Smoothies: Just like in breakfast, smoothies are packed with vitamins and minerals that can provide energy to the body for the rest of the afternoon.

- Eggs: These are not limited to breakfast dishes. Eggs can be hard-boiled or soft-boiled and used as toppings for salads, sandwiches or wraps.

- Fruits: Take them as refreshing desserts that can perk you up during a sleepy lunch hour. The cooling effects as well as the minerals and vitamins can help improve your energy levels and focus.

Dinner

Typically, people eat the most at dinner because it is often the only time of the day when they can really sit down and enjoy a good meal. Breakfast is usually grab-and-go. Lunch may often be a working lunch like eating during a meeting, while working in front of a computer, or on a site visit/inspection. Most people also often have the most proteins for dinner. Carbohydrates are usually light to moderate because the body will not need much energy during the night.

Steaks, chicken, pork, beef, fish and seafood are good ideas for dinner proteins. Grill, steam, bake, sauté, or broil them, and serve over mashed potatoes, wilted greens or fresh salads. Or, use ground meats and sauté them with vegetables like broccoli and root vegetables. Meats are versatile and can be both filling and healthy, if cooked well (without any added unhealthy cooking oil).

Chapter 15

The Healthy Shopping List

Shopping for healthy foods requires knowledge and understanding. It also needs a good plan and a strategy. Before taking a trip to the grocery store, you should have a plan. It would be very helpful to have a weekly menu plan before making a shopping list. This will help in preventing that impulsive grabbing of unhealthy packaged foods in the grocery aisles or grabbing some frozen TV dinners or pizza.

Start at the produce section

When out to shop, head straight to where fresh produce is displayed. Stock up on fruits and vegetables which are rich in most of the things the body needs to achieve health goals such as detoxification, weight loss, revving up metabolism, etc. This strategy accomplishes 2 main things: it fills up the shopping cart/basket leaving little room for unhealthy food choices, and it sets the mind to thinking of what best to pair with these fresh, whole foods. Start by picking at least 6 to 8 different vegetables and about 4 different fruits.

When buying vegetables and fruits, plan ahead. Consider how long these fresh produce will last. Leafy greens should be consumed early into the week before they wilt. Hardier foods like potatoes and other root vegetables can be consumed later. Thin- skinned fruits like berries also won't last long. Foods that have short shelf life must be consumed within a day or two to retain freshness. Also, it will be more practical to buy only the amounts that can be consumed within that period.

Here's a good list to start with when shopping at the produce section:

Greens: These are great whether detoxing, losing weight, building muscles, or improving health. Buy a variety of greens for different flavors and textures. Don't limit greens to lettuce for some crunch in fresh salads. There is a huge selection of green leafy vegetables to choose from. Try some kale, arugula, collard greens, radicchio, spinach, or escarole. To add some crunch, choose greens like broccoli and Brussels sprouts. Wilted greens such as kale and chard are also good additions as side dishes or as a bed for proteins like eggs, fish, chicken or steak. Include fresh herbs for this section, too. Add some coriander leaves, parsley, spring onions and the like. Herbs are rich in healing compounds that can help the body get back on track towards health and healing.

Potatoes: These are a very versatile, healthy carbohydrate source. Potatoes can be baked, steamed, boiled, mashed, etc. A single russet potato contains 150 calories but it nonetheless filling. It also has a high potassium content that helps the body in several ways. Potatoes can be added to various vegetables dishes either mashed or cooked whole. Sweet potatoes are also good to add.

Snack vegetables: while in the produce section, start thinking about to have for snacks. Yes, snacks are not just about opening a bag of chips or eating a box of cookies. The fresh produce section is brimming with healthy snack options. Grab some celery stalks, carrots and cucumbers. Slice them up into sticks and place in snack-size containers. When stressed and looking for some distracting activity, open one and munch on celery and carrot sticks. It distracts, reduces stress and fills up the body, not to mention the various healthy processes the compounds help promote. Other good snack options are bell peppers and jicama, along with any other crunchy, juicy vegetables available.

Berries: Berries are best when they are season. They are sweet and with the highest amount of nutrients, as well as cheap. When not in season, best to look for other fruit options. They'd be not as sweet, and would likely have some artificial chemicals in them. Berries are usually eaten as part of a power breakfast, with oats or as part of a power smoothie. These can be healthy snacks, or a healthier dessert. Stack on berries when in season. Before they become overripe, turn them into jams or preserves. Homemade ones are much healthier because the type and amount of sugar to use can be chosen and controlled to fit into a healthier lifestyle. Also, use of preservatives and other artificial ingredients can be minimized.

Apples: These are perfect snacks that can come in handy at any time. They make perfect desserts, too. Keep the skin on because it's where most of the fibers and the other phytonutrients are found. To keep things more interesting, dip apple slices in almond or peanut butter. For a great take on an apple dessert, roast some apples and sprinkle with a mixture of brown sugar and cinnamon. It's decadent yet still healthy.

Walk to the protein section

After the produce, go to the proteins section. Just buy 3 to 4 proteins. They may be stored in the freezer for a week or so, but it's best to buy fresh ones every week. Also, meat proteins should be limited, as the best proteins are still from plants (such as lentils and beans).

Ground meat: This is a very versatile meat ingredient. When shopping, grab a package of lean ground turkey or chicken. This can be made into a healthy burger for snack or quick lunch. Or, add to pasta sauce and pour over whole grain pasta. There are endless options for lean ground meats. These are also perfect backup protein stock. Ground meats are often on sale so buy a few extras and store properly in the freezer. They keep for up to 3 months. When out of options, just thaw one and cook with some vegetables.

Pork: This kind of meat has been pushed to the side for years because of all the bad raps about pork fat, belly, bacon, and all pig products. These were considered the epitome of what unhealthy is. But, people should be aware that there are healthy cuts of pork. Try pork tenderloin or boneless pork chops to shake things up a bit from the usual chicken breasts.

Seafood: Shellfish and fish are full of essential fats, low in calories, and rich in various minerals. Experts recommend eating fish at least 2 times each week to reap health benefits. Go for salmon, tuna, mackerel, sardines and trout. Also, try having shellfish like mussels and clams.

At this point, the grocery cart should be almost filled by now. And, meals for an entire week should already be shaping and almost complete. The next few sections will include just as few items to keep meals tasty and interesting.

A quick stop at the frozen foods sections

Not everything in this section is bad. It has a few good choices, too. For instance, frozen vegetables and fruits out of season can still be enjoyed. However, there will be issues on taste and flavor. These may not be as delicious as fresh ones. Also, freezing can destroy the nutrients. Choose items that have been freeze-dried or flash frozen. Any damage to the nutrients is minimal. But, if fresh ones are available, get the fresh ones.

 Sorbet is another good reason to visit the frozen food section. These are made with fresh fruits and with little dairy. Choose ones with only a small percentage of milk or cream, and with little to no added sugars. Sorbet makes for healthy desserts and snacks to help satisfy sweet cravings without worrying about sugars and lactose.

Visit the dairy section

While some people may need to limit their intake of dairy, there are a few items in this section that can be added to the grocery cart.

Eggs: Eggs are perfect protein, fat, mineral, and vitamin sources. This is an excellent protein source that's very versatile and easy to prepare. Make some vegetable omelet for breakfast and it's already packed with all t eh nutrients like protein, carbs, fats, minerals and vitamins. Boil some eggs and add to salads for lunch. Poach some and eat as mid-afternoon snack. Add to some olive oil and make a protein-packed healthy dressing over grilled steak or fish for dinner.

Cheese: Get the fresh cheeses as dairy or natural seasoning for food. To add some saltiness in vegetable salads, add some crumbled feta cheese or Parmesan shavings. Cube some feta and add to a medley of fruits for snacks. A little goes a long way and cheeses can help add more healthy flavors to food any time.

Yogurt: Greek yogurt is rich in probiotics that have great benefits for health. It makes for a great breakfast and for snacks. Top with berries and fresh fruits and the day is set for a greats start. Greek yogurt can also be used as a base for dressings and dips.

And lastly, grab some good whole grains. These are filling and great substitutes to white rice and pasta. Get some quinoa and turn them into a power-packed breakfast meal with berries or other fruits. Barley, faro, and bulgur are also grain choices. These grains can be combined with any leftover meats or vegetable dishes and make a warm salad for lunch or dinner. Toss in some herbs and wrap in corn tortilla or in some lettuce leaves for a healthy filling lunch. Add some dressing and herbs for a great healthy side dish.

Chapter 16

Low Sugar Recipes

Sugar is almost always present in food. Carbohydrates can be converted into sugar, as well as fats and proteins. What can be done to reduce sugar intake is to avoid the use of added sugars. Learn to use the natural sweetness in certain foods. Natural sweeteners such as honey should be used in moderation. Other condiments can be used to flavor food. Also, avoid using refined sugar.

Here are a few recipes to try that significantly reduces the use of added sugars and ingredients that have high sugar contents:

Turkey, cheese and spinach wrap

This recipe has less than 1 gram of sugar in it and it comes from the cheese. No added sugars but filling and satisfying.

Ingredients:

- Turkey sausage links, make sure to get one that has no added sugars and with less salt

- ¼ cup of shredded Cheddar cheese, reduced-fat version

- 1 piece 8-inch whole wheat tortilla

- 1 cup of spinach leaves

Heat the tortilla in a pan until softened. Set aside. In the same pan, sauté sliced sausage links in a little olive oil. Set aside and drain on a paper towel. Arrange the turkey wrap. Place spinach leaves on the tortilla. Top with sautéed sausage and cheese. Wrap securely.

Caesar salad

Most store-bought condiments, dips, and dressings are full of sugar and salt. Learn to make your own condiments at home to control the sugar and salt that go into them. Caesar salad dressing is among the most versatile dressings. When you are on a healthy diet, salads are going to be the main food on your plate. That would mean using dressings on a fairly constant basis.

Ingredients:

- 1 medium-sized egg

- 1 clove of garlic, finely minced

- 1 ½ teaspoon of anchovy paste (to serve as salt substitute and for added flavor)

- ½ teaspoon of Dijon mustard

- 2 tablespoons of lemon juice, freshly squeezed

- ¼ teaspoon of Worcestershire sauce

- 2 tablespoons of olive oil

- ¼ cup of freshly grated Parmesan

Place all ingredients except the olive oil and cheese in a small bowl and whisk until smooth and even. Slowly add olive oil in a thin and steady stream while continuously whisking. When smooth, add parmesan cheese and stir until well combined. Use as dressing over salads or on sandwiches.

Mashed potatoes

Mashed potatoes are going to be one of the main dishes in most meals. It is a better substitute to rice or pasta. It is a great source of healthy complex carbohydrates that will not cause any spikes in blood sugar levels. Traditional mashed potatoes use heavy cream which often has added sugars. By substituting heavy cream with buttermilk, the nutrients are improved and calories and sugars are reduced.

Ingredients:

- 2 pounds of potatoes, cubed, skin on because it is where most of the fibers are

- 1 tablespoon of salt

- 1 cup of buttermilk, low fat version

- 1 ½ tablespoon of organic butter

- 2 tablespoons of chives, chopped, for garnish

Place the potatoes in a large pot. Fill with enough water to cover the potatoes. Place over medium high heat setting and bring it to a boil. Cook until potatoes become tender, which would take about 20 minutes. Set aside to slightly cool. Warm the buttermilk in a saucepan over low heat setting. Be careful with overheating the buttermilk. Set aside when heated through. Drain excess liquid from the potatoes. Mash the potatoes in a large bowl. Carefully pour the buttermilk into the potatoes. Stir to mix well. Season according to taste with pepper and salt. Finish the mashed potato by mixing in the butter, serve with a sprinkle of chopped chives. Serve with meats, seafood, fish or poultry.

Spicy Asian dressing

As an alternative to Caesar dressing or to keep meals more interesting, try an Asian dressing. This can also be drizzled over meats, poultry, or seafood for added flavors. This recipe has chilies, which can irritate the gut lining in sensitive people. Omit this if this is the case. If not, chili can help in revving up metabolism and speed up fat burning.

Ingredients:

- 1 tablespoon fish sauce

- 1 tablespoon soy sauce

- 1 teaspoon rice vinegar

- 1 tablespoon fresh lime juice

- 1/2 teaspoon olive oil

- 1/2 to 1 whole jalapeño, according to preference

- 2 cloves garlic, minced

Place all ingredients in a medium bowl. Mix well and drizzle over salads or over cooked meats.

Chapter 17

Living a Green Life

Living a green life further helps you in achieving a perfectly healthy body. Living a green life means reducing use of and exposure to anything and everything artificial. This kind of lifestyle helps to reduce toxin exposure that can create imbalances in the body and increase the risk of contracting certain diseases.

Remove toxins in the home

The home is great place to start when making changes towards living a green life. There are so many toxins in the home, if one knows where to look. Start with the cleaning products. Even the dishwashing liquid used in cleaning pots, pans, plates and utensils is a potential source of toxins that enter the body and create health problems. The various cleaning agents leave chemical residues on surfaces even when rinsed well with water. These residues can get into the skin, eyes, and food. Once inside the body, they can set off negative cellular processes that interfere with the body's natural balance. Throw these away and choose certified toxic-free, green products.

Check body and personal care products

Another major potential source of toxins is care products. Shampoos, lotions, creams, gels, and soaps are all potentially filled with toxins. These may come in the form of emulsifiers, stabilizers, fragrances, colorants, and preservatives in these products. Choose products made from organic products, with natural fragrances. Any product that has a long list of ingredients or contains ingredients that's difficult to pronounce, it's potentially toxic.

Clean the air

Pollutants in the air are another major source of toxin. While it isn't possible to clean outside air, it can be purified inside the home. Plant trees around the house or cultivate some plants and place them around the house. Plants are natural air cleaners that can help in reducing exposure to air pollutants.

Avoid processed foods

Again, the effect of processed foods is never good. The ingredients have been heavily altered that the body can no longer make any good use of them. Opt for fresh, locally produced foods instead. Local produce are least likely to be treated with chemicals because they do not need to travel far.

Choose organic

Organic means materials and food that have not been exposed to toxic chemicals such as preservatives, insecticides, artificial fertilizers and pesticides. Choose organically grown fresh produce. Also, meats, meat products and dairy should come from grass-fed, free-range animal sources.

Chapter 18

Getting the Best Supplements

Supplements are important because these are not usually found in large amounts in the food we eat. One would have to eat tons of certain foods in order to get enough of these "extra nutrients". The good news is that supplements are available. Just check with a doctor first before taking because these supplements may interfere with certain medications and treatments. Also, some of these supplements may cause more problems if taken without a doctor's advice.

Branched chain amino acid (BCAA)

Branched chain amino acids are popular among people who wish to build muscles. It is also a great supplement to reduce muscle soreness that usually occurs during workouts. A research study conducted at the UK's University of Birmingham has shown that BCAA supplements can significantly reduce exercise-induced muscle soreness. Another study conducted in Brazil showed that taking BCAA reduces fatigue and increases the rate of fat burning in the body.

Creatinine

Creatinine is a natural molecule in the body needed for muscle function. Supplementing can help in improving, building and strengthening lean muscles. One study found that taking creatinine supplements increases the levels of IGF-1 (insulin-like growth factor-1) in the body. This molecule has anabolic effects in the body that enhances the effects of resistance training.

Conjugated linoleic acid (CLA)

CLA or conjugated linoleic acid contains omega-3 fatty acids. Researchers have found that CLA can accelerate fat burning in the body while preserving muscles.

Glutamine

Glutamine supplements reduce inflammation in the body. It also helps in fighting off infections. One study in Italy found that glutamine supplements can stimulate muscle growth, too. Glutamine is a natural compound in the body that regulates glycogen (stored sugars in the muscles). By boosting glycogen, muscles have enhanced performance and growth.

Chapter 19

The Best Exercise for Overall Health

Exercise is important in achieving a healthy body. It does not have to be a special gym class or take hours in day. It just means moving different muscle groups at a time. It can be as simple as walking 2 to 3 blocks a day or climbing 2 flights of stairs instead of taking the elevator or escalator.

How to get more exercise

One of the biggest excuses in not exercising is lack of time. Most people are too busy with work and daily responsibilities that they feel they have no time to exercise. The truth is anyone can squeeze in enough time for exercise even in the middle of a busy day—as long as one is willing to get some exercise.

One bit of good news for people who can't seem to find time to exercise is a study conducted in New Zealand. In this study, it was determined that exercise can be performed on a "snack basis". Most people think that when they exercise, they need to do so for at least 30 minutes at a time in order to gain the benefits. But in this study, spending 3 10-minute exercises per day can achieve the same benefits. It's like having a "breakfast, lunch, dinner" sort of exercise. This kind of routine is already effective in lowering the levels of glucose in the blood and in burning fat all day long.

This type of exercise is also known as short circuit sessions. The routine targets the core that effectively blasts stubborn fats. The best time to start mini workouts is early in the morning. A study showed that exposure to the early morning to noonday sun helps in reducing weight gain. Exposure alone is enough to get this benefit, without any relation to activity level, age or caloric intake. The body is connected to nature and the morning light is synced to the body's own circadian rhythm. Exposure to morning light jumpstarts the metabolism, acting like a natural alarm that wakes up the body. It is also believed to undercut the fat genes in the body. With exposure to the morning light, the body is already burning calories from its fat stores rather than from what was eaten for breakfast. Time a short exercise and calories burned will surely be much higher. In fact, people who tried mini circuits (10-minute workout) in the morning sun experienced increase in heart rates a few moments into the workout.

Chapter 20

How to Prevent Diseases

Disease prevention is also important in living a better, healthier life. Infections can cause imbalances in the body. Together with diseases, infections can damage tissues that can set off imbalances. It is equally important to protect the body against diseases.

Drugs are not the only ones to use in preventing diseases. In fact, drugs can be a source of toxins and stress that places the body out of balance. Limit your intake of drugs and always take these only with advice from a doctor. Avoid taking any medication that isn't prescribed by a doctor and should only be taken within the prescribed period.

The best ways to prevent diseases include the following:

- Get enough sleep. Adults tend to take sleep for granted, especially nighttime sleep. A lot of people think that sleep is sleep no matter when it happens. There are lots of studies that show nighttime sleep is very different to daytime sleep. The body is naturally designed to rest, replenish and reset at night during sleep. Daytime sleep will not produce these same effects. In fact, daytime sleepers will have more problem in regulating metabolism and hormones because the body is forced to reverse its natural schedule. Aim to get more sleep at night.

- Hydrate. Water is important. The body is composed of at least 70% water, and each cellular process requires water. Excretion requires water, too. So make sure to drink at least 2 liters of water each day. Drink more if the weather is hot, when sweating, or when exercising. Always keep a bottle of water on hand. Drinking water can instantly make the body feel better, too. If feeling low in energy, sluggish, or a little under the weather, you should drink lots of water. This can help in restoring the body's strength against any infection or disease.

- Supplement. Vitamins and minerals from multivitamin supplements can help in strengthening immunity and fighting off infections. The body is always exposed to pathogens and strengthening the immune system is very important to prevent getting sick.

Aside from these major steps, disease prevention includes eating well-balanced meals and engaging in regular exercise. Avoiding exposure is also crucial. Avoid crowds and stay away from known polluted areas. If such can't be avoided, you should take the necessary steps to strengthen your immune system.

Conclusion

To achieve optimum results, the healthy changes discussed in this book should be sustained. Dieting, detoxing, weight loss, and muscle building are not short-term processes; they all have to become part of an overall healthy lifestyle.

Start making these changes today and you will be well on your way to a healthier and more enjoyable life.

Don't forget to tell others about this book so that they, too, can be healthier.

Good luck in achieving your health goals! And if you enjoyed this book and it was able to help you in any way, please leave me a nice review at Amazon, I would really appreciate it.

Melinda

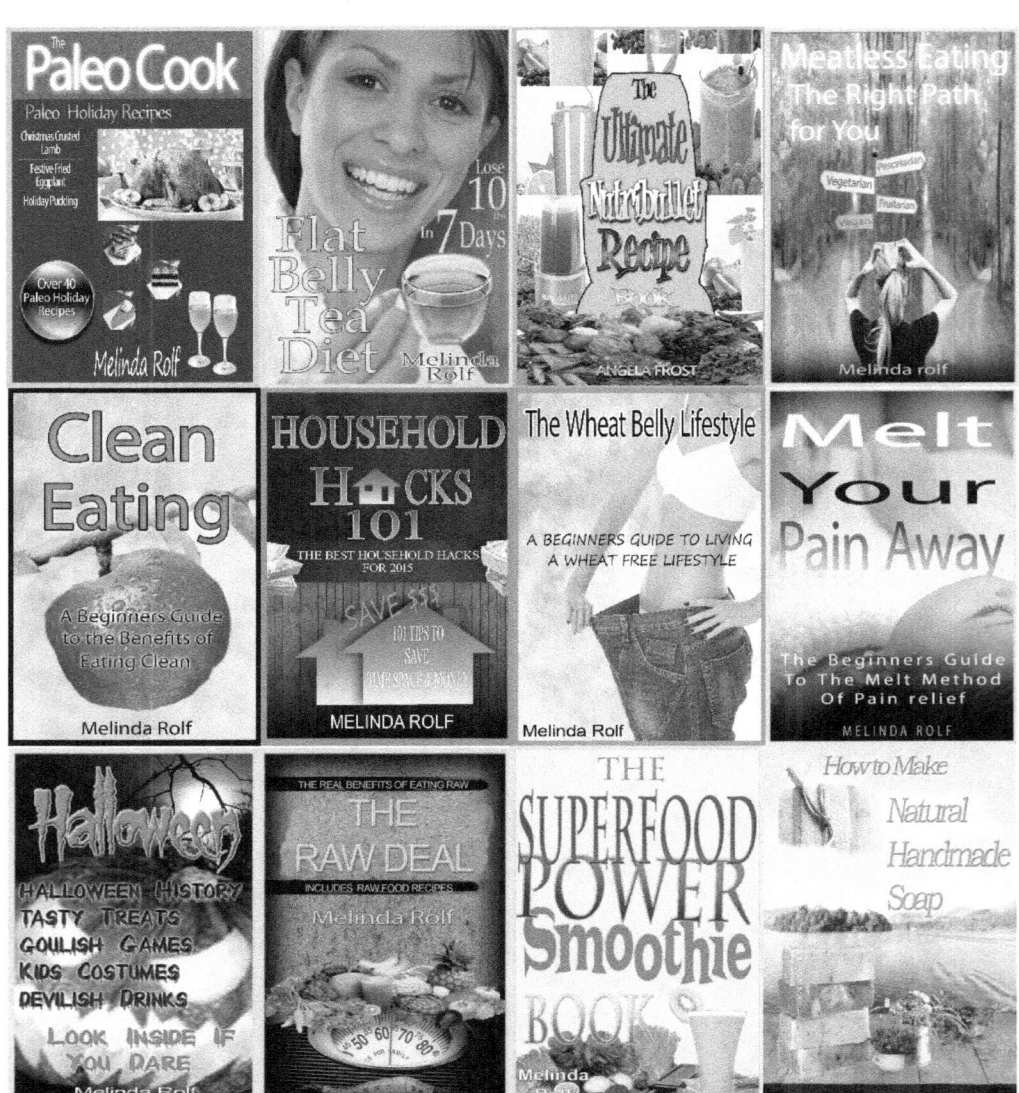

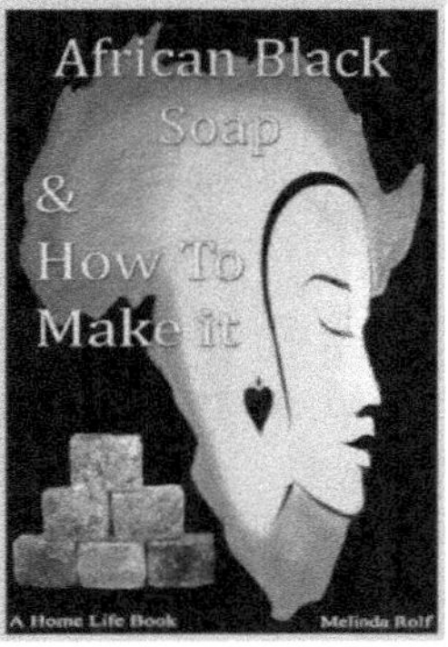

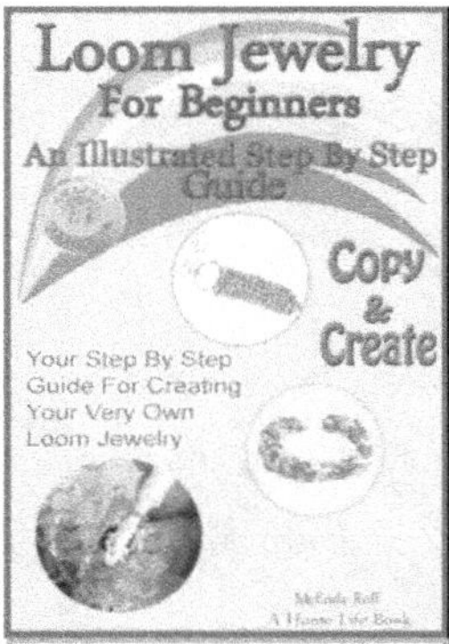

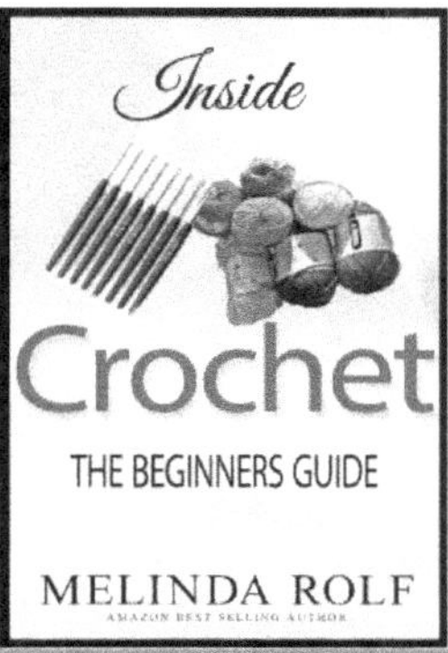

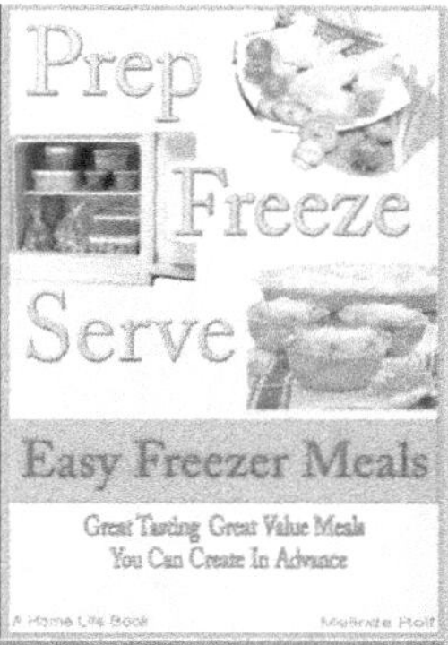

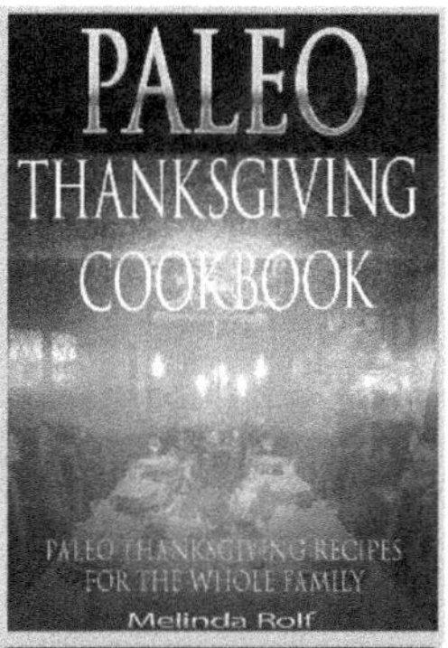

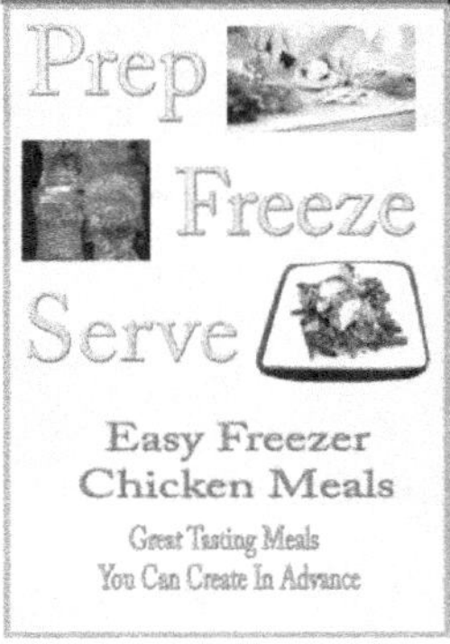

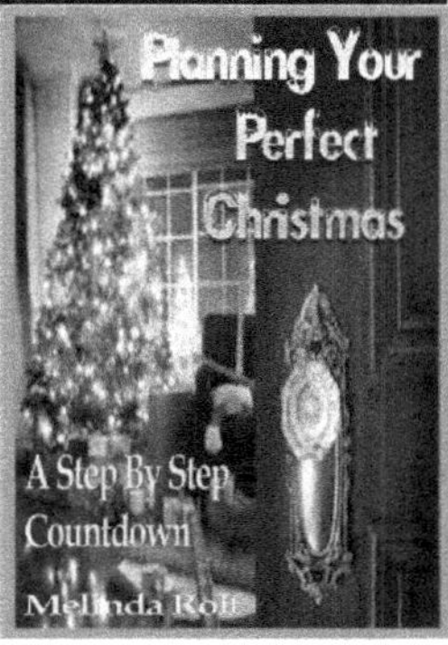

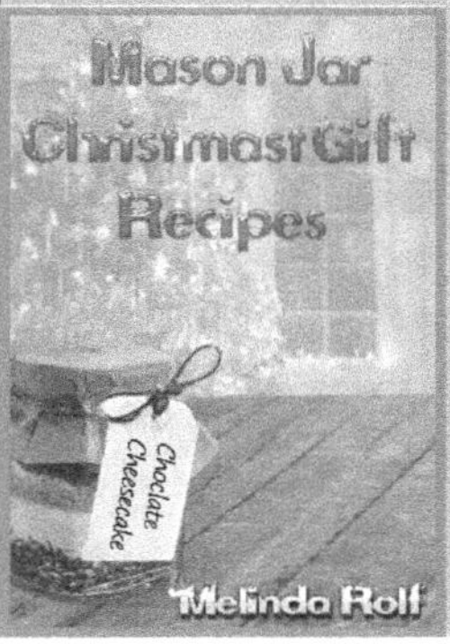

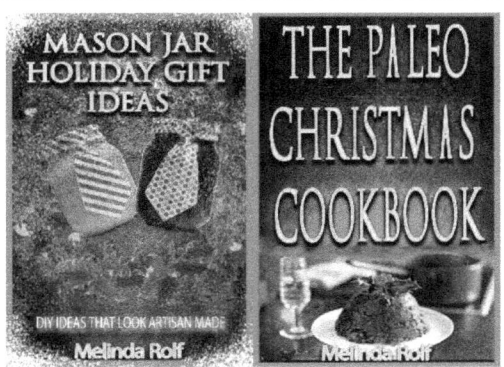

See All eQuivia Books

Available at Amazon and other fine stores in e-book and paperback format

About the Author

Melinda (AKA Angela Frost) is an Amazon best selling author and..... health nut, tea lover, soapmaker, cooking and freezing expert, crocheterer, and mom of three

Melinda loves anything to do with the home and the home life which is why she has taken her love and knowledge and turned them in a series of books called "The Home Life Series" In these books you will find recipes, crochet patterns, freezing tips, soap recipes, Holday recipes, Paleo and Diabetic cookbooks, smoothies, tea diets, and so much more.

She hopes you will enjoy them and that thery are able to help you in some way. And if so, please leave us a nice review, we would really appreciate it.

Melinda lives with her husband, 3 children 2 dogs, a cat, and a yellow bellied turtle in Swanville, Maine

Like me on Facebook

Follow me on Twitter

Visit my website

www.ingramcontent.com/pod-product-compliance
Lightning Source LLC
Chambersburg PA
CBHW070436290526
45791CB00005B/1994